PAIN, SUFFERING AND HEALING

Pain, Suffering and Healing

insights and understanding

Edited by

PETER WEMYSS-GORMAN

Retired Consultant in Anaesthesia and Pain Medicine,
Princes Royal Hospital, Haywards Heath, UK

Foreword by

JOHN D LOESER

Professor Emeritus of Neurological Surgery and Anesthesiology and
Pain Medicine, University of Washington, Seattle, WA, USA

Radcliffe Publishing
London • New York

Radcliffe Publishing Ltd
33–41 Dallington Street
London
EC1V 0BB
UK

www.radcliffepublishing.com

Electronic catalogue and worldwide online ordering facility.

British Library Cataloguing in Publication Data

A catalogue record for this book is available from the British Library.

ISBN-13: 978 184619 326 2

The paper used for the text pages of this book is FSC® certified. FSC (The Forest Stewardship Council®) is an international network to promote responsible management of the world's forests.

Typeset by Phoenix Photosetting, Chatham, Kent, UK
Cover designed by Andrew Magee Design, Banbury, Oxon, UK
Printed and bound by TJI Digital, Padstow, Cornwall, UK

Contents

To my wife Jean, with thanks for the hours she spent helping to turn my prolix phraseology into readable English, and for her unfailing love and support through all the long years when it seemed that this project would never reach fruition.

Royalties from this book will be donated to Freedom from Torture, formerly the Medical Foundation for the Care of Victims of Torture.

Foreword

Although modern medicine has made some progress in the treatment of pain, we have clearly fared less well against suffering. Indeed, the contemporary push to make healthcare providers more 'efficient' has put great pressure on primary care practitioners to see more patients per hour and has minimised the opportunities to deal with the patient's suffering, as well as many of the other effects of pain. Listening to a patient's narrative takes time, and suffering can only be addressed through the patient's narrative. Biomedicine has no place for suffering; a biopsychosocial perspective is the underpinning for this book. Our predecessors thought of the nervous system as hard-wired, and functioning in a stimulus–response organisation. Pain was the by-product of a disease state; treatment of the disease should eliminate pain and the associated suffering. We now know that the nervous system has enormous flexibility and that all sensory inputs are strongly modulated. We also know that eye witnesses are notoriously unreliable; a patient is the epitome of an eye witness. What we experience is coloured by our past experiences and the anticipated consequences. The placebo response demonstrates this with clarity. Unfortunately, there are still those who think the old way about pain and suffering, and that is why this book deserves a wide audience.

Cassell defined suffering as the threat to the physical or psychological integrity of the individual.[1] Healthcare providers have, all too often, looked only at the physical aspects of suffering and have overlooked the psychological issues. In the past, other types of providers dealt with suffering; but in the 21st century in the developed countries, they are sparse. Religious answers appear to be less satisfying; people want happiness and freedom from suffering in this life, not one yet to come. Physicians are now expected to identify and resolve suffering in the absence of training to do this and without time to interact with the patient. What was swept under the rug is now publicly discussed. The healthcare provider is expected to deal with issues that used to be brought to religious leaders or grandmothers. Healthcare is going to have to broaden the approach to patients who suffer from chronic pain. Education of physicians and nurses must be expanded to deal with issues such as suffering.

Chronic pain is an existential condition that probably will never be resolved by biomedicine. It is the suffering engendered by chronic pain that mandates that healthcare providers address the issues. Suffering cannot be found in a laboratory test or imaging study; it is only observable by communicating with the sufferer. The 11 chapters in this book approach this conundrum from vastly different perspectives, some highly personal and others broadly social. Membership in the Special Interest Group of the British Pain Society for Philosophy and Ethics has stimulated the authors to create a text for both professionals and lay persons. Issues such as the interface between the physician and the pharmaceutical industry are also presented. Each chapter author describes a facet of the problems of suffering and some of the available paths to recovery. There are no simple answers to complex questions, and there is no single way to enlightenment. It is always the patient who must do the work to resolve his or her suffering; the healthcare provider can only act as a guide and provide encouragement. The authors of the chapters in this book have provided a collection of narratives which readers can use to pursue their own truths.

John D Loeser, MD
Professor Emeritus, of Neurological Surgery and Anesthesiology
and Pain Medicine, University of Washington, Seattle, WA, USA
July 2011

REFERENCE

1   Cassell EJ. *The Nature of Suffering and the Goals of Medicine*. New York: Oxford University Press; 1991.

Preface

Pain and suffering have been a major preoccupation of philosophers for millennia and more has been written on the subject than almost any other. It may well be asked: what, then, is the need for yet another book on philosophy and suffering? Aside from the fact that no book can ever provide the last word on, or even a comprehensive guide to, such a vast and complex subject, this book is unusual in that it is written mainly by professionals working with suffering people. Although this of course includes virtually the whole medical and allied professions, the last half century has seen the emergence of a whole new specialism engaged specifically in the treatment and management of pain. Daily contact with people in pain and the frequent difficulty of providing adequate relief inevitably raises questions that go beyond the clinical, which this book is intended to address in ways which are both thoughtful and relevant to real life in the consulting room. Although the readership is anticipated to be mainly professional, there are countless people who have to live with suffering, either their own or that of others, and are seeking meaning in it. Some may justifiably feel let down by the medical professions, and will be encouraged to know that there are many of us who are also struggling for understanding; and may also find this book helpful. Critics may detect in my own contributions some lack of clarity as to whether I am addressing health professionals or patients. I would contend that this reflects a growing conviction of the relationship between the two as that of partners, and the vital importance of dialogue between them in the search for mutual understanding.

THE SPECIAL INTEREST GROUP OF THE BRITISH PAIN SOCIETY FOR PHILOSOPHY AND ETHICS

At the Vienna Congress of the International Association for the Study of Pain in 1999 we had been, as always on these occasions, bombarded with science and the message from the multi-million dollar drug industry that no effort or expense could ever be spared in the battle to defeat pain.

Feeling slightly battered by all this, a colleague and I had taken a day off. We both admitted to feeling quite depressed by the relatively little obvious relevance of much of what we had been hearing to the everyday realities of dealing with distressed human beings in the pain clinic. We recalled how we had first met some 20 years previously at a conference designed to bring 'pain' and 'hospice' doctors together, in the tranquil surroundings of Scargill House in the heart of the Yorkshire Dales, and it occurred to us that it might be useful to try to arrange some sort of meeting there to reflect on what we were trying to achieve and should realistically be expecting to achieve, and how to accept and cope with our relative impotence in the face of so much unrelieved pain.

And so in the summer of 2001 a group of doctors, nurses, psychologists and others working with people in pain got together at Scargill House to tackle some of these questions – not perhaps expecting to find answers but at least to share some of our perplexities and anxieties. This conference, entitled The Inevitability of Pain?, was intended as a 'one-off' but the need for a forum for further discussion about such things became immediately apparent and has resulted in a series of annual gatherings. In recognition of the importance of this activity, the core group was recognised in 2004 as a Special Interest Group of the British Pain Society.

Several features have made these meetings different. Besides their unusual subject matter, they have been designed to maximise participation by the audience, and the remit of speakers is to stimulate rather than to inform the debate which, both in full session and informal conversation, takes up a major proportion of the time. The venues, retreat centres in the Yorkshire Dales, Leicestershire and the Lake District, are in areas of famed natural beauty and provide an atmosphere particularly conducive to contemplation and reflection, and to the physical and spiritual recreation so much needed by people wearied by their daily work with human pain and distress.

So much of value has come out of these meetings that we felt it imperative to try to share it with a wider audience. And so the idea of this book evolved. Selection has been difficult and dependant in part on availability and willingness of potential authors; inevitably much of merit has been omitted. Every year since this book began its long gestation more material worthy of inclusion has emerged, and there is already enough for a second volume! Although all the authors have given talks on the same lines at our meetings, these chapters are new and may involve some modification of earlier views, influenced not only by subsequent thoughts but also by the discussion which followed their presentation.

Peter Wemyss-Gorman
July 2011

Introduction

THE DEVELOPMENT OF PAIN MEDICINE

Although pain is, and presumably always has been, the most common presenting complaint in all who consult their doctors, pain medicine as a specialty only emerged in the late 1940s, mainly as the inspiration of John Bonica of Seattle. His seminal work *The Management of Pain* appeared in 1953,[1] and he established the world's first multidisciplinary pain clinic in 1960. Since then there has been an exponential increase in the number of people involved. At the first meeting of the Intractable Pain Society of Great Britain and Northern Ireland in 1967 there were 17 doctors – virtually all the people in the UK working in this field; 10 years later there were still only about 300 members. Now, membership of the British Pain Society stands at nearly 1700, and the International Association for the Study of Pain has more than 7000 members in 106 countries. What started as almost exclusively the domain of anaesthetists has become truly multidisciplinary and encompasses many other specialisms and professions including neurology, psychology, nursing, occupational therapy and physiotherapy. In the UK the number of pain clinics has increased from a dozen or so in the early 1970s to the present day when there is one in nearly every hospital, and there is a similar situation in most affluent countries. This huge expansion of clinical activity has been paralleled by a similar growth in research in neurophysiology, psychology and pharmacology, as well as in clinical medicine. There are at least 26 English-language journals devoted to pain research and practice, and many more in other languages.

Our knowledge about the mechanisms in the brain and nervous system that underlie the conscious experience of pain has increased enormously (*see* Further reading on page xix). Research into the amazing complexities of the mechanisms of pain perception has led us ever deeper, from whole organisms to systems, from systems to cells and from cells to molecules. Arguably the most important aspect of all this has been the realisation that the nervous system is not 'hard-wired', with events in one part of it, such as stimulation of pain receptors beneath the skin, always evoking the same responses in the same parts of the brain. This picture has been replaced by the recognition of 'plastic' changes in the function of the pathways between body and brain and in the brain itself in different circumstances, so that what reaches consciousness is a product of many different influences. It could be said, however, that although the amount of *information* about the mind-boggling complexities of this has multiplied many times the degree to which this has improved our *understanding* is another matter. To dismiss all the research as irrelevant to understanding human pain and useless in its relief would be absurd, but there are problems. The bulk of research has of necessity been reductionist, and despite the efforts of writers such as the late Patrick Wall, rebuilding the pieces into a comprehensible whole which is relevant to human suffering has not always been easy.

Science is extremely good at answering questions that begin with 'how', such as 'How are warning signals of injury conducted from the outside of the body to the brain and consciousness?', but sometimes less helpful with 'why' questions, such as 'Why do innocent people suffer?'.

Alongside all the research has been the pharmaceutical industry, which has spent countless billions in the search for better drugs for relieving pain. There has long been the expectation that any day now we would see the promised breakthrough from basic science to improved therapeutics, and there have been many promising developments, but spin-off in terms of new drugs and interventions has on the whole so far been rather disappointing. (Although we do at least understand the limitations of existing ones rather better.)

There are indeed some areas, notably the palliation of cancer pain, where the picture has improved out of all recognition. Joint replacement surgery has made a huge contribution to the reduction of human suffering (a fact sometimes overlooked by pain doctors who see only orthopaedic surgeons' failures). Nevertheless there are many other areas, notably chronic back pain and neuropathic pain (pain arising within the nervous system), where cure is rare, prolonged relief unusual and the best that can usually be achieved is some reduction in pain intensity and improvement in limitation of activity – and sometimes not even this.

In some ways the most important advance has been the recognition of the reality that the experience of suffering involves a complex interaction of physical and emotional influences, and a re-emergence of the ancient concept of healing the whole person. Many patients are caught up in a vicious circle of depression, anxiety and limitation of activity as much due to fear of pain as pain itself. The lives of many have been transformed by pain management programmes, where teams of psychologists, physiotherapists, occupational therapists and specialist nurses work together to enable patients to recognise and deal with self-defeating thought processes and inappropriate behaviour patterns. But not everybody can be helped even in this way.

Few of the benefits of modern pain medicine, limited as they are, have devolved to large parts of the world where economic and medical resources are poor and even the most basic health needs are inadequately catered for. Indeed it could be said that all the combined efforts of all the pain professionals in the world have done little more than scratch the surface of the totality of human suffering, and show little sign of ever doing much better.

These realities are only too familiar to pain professionals, but rarely faced in our conventional clinical and scientific meetings. There is so much to be learnt – so great the pressure to improve our understanding of pain mechanisms, learn of new drugs and improve techniques – that there is rarely time to stand back, so to speak, and reflect on what we can realistically hope to achieve, or even be trying to achieve. We are so busy trying to answer 'how' questions, we fail to address the 'why' questions that our patients tax us with. We tell them that they must learn to accept their pain but fail to face and accept our own impotence to relieve it.

A FORETASTE

The inspiration for the first gathering of the Special Interest Group of the British Pain Society for Philosophy and Ethics in the summer of 2001 derived in part from an article in *Pain Reviews* by Willy Notcutt entitled 'The Tao of Pain'.[2] Willy presented it at that meeting and Chapter 1 is a revised and extended version of this. He explores the changes in thinking about pain and its treatment over the last three decades in the terms of Fritz Capra's *Tao of Physics*,[3] which brings together physics and Eastern mysticism and parallels the progression from simple through more and more complex science to mystery, which the search for understanding suffering involves, and questions the common perception of pain as an enemy which must be defeated by the most aggressive means available, rather than trying to reach a deeper understanding of the meaning of pain for our patients.

The words 'pain' and 'suffering' are often used either together or more or less interchangeably, and I plead guilty to having done so already. But they are not synonymous. They are both of course very difficult to define. As the much-quoted IASP definition suggests, pain is usually associated with tissue damage, and although it is a subjective experience and involves 'mental' and emotional processes it is still largely a 'body' thing, and can at least in part be understood by studying the nervous system. It is shared by 'lower' animals and even chronic pain can be looked at in the context of evolutionary biology. Suffering is much more elusive. Although it is perhaps most often associated with 'physical' pain, it has many other sources both within and outside the individual. And although it is manifested as distress, sadness, depression and anxiety the whole seems more than the sum of its parts. It could be said to be a 'spiritual' thing. It appears to have no adaptive function – and indeed would seem to be in a different category from things that do. (I realise that

I am in danger of subscribing to a 'pain/suffering' dualism which would be as misleading as 'mind/body' dualism and it is clear that in both cases the concepts are inextricably entwined.) Pain can often be relieved by the doctor as technician, but suffering demands that he fulfils his role as a healer. Suffering robs us of choice, and in Chapter 2 Michael Bavidge explores the distinction between pain and suffering in the context of the influence of suffering on choice and autonomy.

Suffering raises apparently unanswerable questions all beginning with 'why' and although it challenges the concept of a God of love religions have evolved in large part to try to give it meaning. In Chapter 3 Michael Hare Duke examines historically changing attitudes to pain and its relief and beliefs such as that the divine purpose involves personal growth through suffering. He shows that such questions, which have no clear and easy answers, have always been addressed through poetry and myth rather than by logical argument.

Readers may have gained the impression so far that our deliberations in the meetings of the group have been somewhat 'cerebral' and divorced from the realities of everyday clinical practice, but this would be a misleading picture. The participants are mostly those whose daily work is essentially clinical and practical. Their first priority is to try to relieve pain. But as well as the limitations of our ability to achieve this there are many ethical and other dilemmas involved in the practice of pain medicine which give rise to much uncertainty and anxiety. These include such issues as the prescription of drugs of potential abuse for patients who are vulnerable to this problem. Difficulties also arise in the relationship between the medical profession and the drug industry. While acknowledging the great contribution of the latter to the provision of drugs for pain, it has to be recognised that the astronomical costs of research and development may lead to inappropriate pressures on clinical researchers and doubtful marketing methods, with inappropriate inducements for doctors to prescribe new products. Willy Notcutt discusses this in Chapter 4.

Growing recognition of the value and importance of pain medicine has led to demand outstripping provision, and in many areas waiting lists for pain clinics are far too long and progression through allied professions such as physiotherapy and psychology far too slow. The Pain Society and more recently the Chronic Pain Policy Coalition have long and vigorously campaigned for better governmental recognition of the inadequacy of provision for pain services. But however repugnant it may seem, resources will for the foreseeable future have to be rationed to maximise benefit to the maximum number of sufferers. This necessitates a clear perception of what pain services are actually for. Much of the work, for instance, involves interventions such as injections for back pain which may provide a period of blessed relief but are rarely curative and arguably may only put off the evil hour of accepting the pain and learning to live productive lives in spite of it. Both individual clinical decision making and resource allocation are supposed to be grounded in evidence-based medicine but the application of this to such a complex and unquantifiable a problem as human suffering is rarely straightforward. In Chapter 5 Ian Yellowlees looks at changing concepts of pain management and the need for correcting unrealistic expectations of both patients and referring doctors of what pain clinics can achieve. He argues that the traditional roles of the doctor to treat the patient and of the patient passively to accept this needs to be replaced by a partnership in which the patient also has responsibilities and work to do. But there are patients with a tendency to dependency who may not benefit from this approach and for whom repeated interventions may arguably be appropriate. Currently the type of management a patient receives may depend more on the doctor's prejudices and enthusiasms than the patient's individual needs, and the need for re-examination of the role of pain services and remodelling of the way they work, with a clear idea of what they are for, is overwhelming.

Pain clinicians and indeed most health professionals will be only too familiar with the picture of the patient who arrives with notes several inches thick, a sorry story of consultations and hospital admissions over many years for a variety of complaints mainly involving pain, but with a definitive diagnosis of a specific illness hardly ever having been proved. Such patients have become highly dependent, demanding of repeated physical interventions, and are often indignantly dismissive of any suggestion that they might be helped by a psychological approach. Continuing Ian Yellowlees' theme, in Chapter 6 Diana Brighouse suggests that pain clinics should be offering such patients more than either repeated injections to keep them happy or yet another rejection to add to their unhappy catalogue. She examines the inadequacies of the reductionist approach which has dominated modern scientific medicine for dealing with the complexities of human suffering, and maintains that the inherent problems of some patients are compounded by the dualistic mindset of doctors who assume that if symptoms cannot be explained or treated on a biomedical model they must be psychological, and if they reject or do not respond to simple psychological measures such as cognitive behavioural therapy, they are beyond hope. Such patients can, however, be helped by a long-term reparative relationship with a therapist who over many hours and months tries to enable them to acknowledge and deal with deep-seated problems which frequently include a history of childhood abuse.

One of the phenomena which have long puzzled and tantalised both brain scientists and pain clinicians is that of the placebo response. Its power is undeniable; it was indeed the main therapeutic tool of our medical ancestors which we arguably should not discard. It is, however, often regarded as a nuisance by people trying to design objective assessments of drugs and other therapies, and presents ethical difficulties in this context. Trying deliberately to exploit it by encouraging unrealistic expectations of the efficacy of a treatment may well be regarded as dishonest. I explore these fascinating but difficult paradoxes in Chapter 7.

The inclination to try to prevent or relieve suffering in one's fellows would appear to be part of human nature. But there is a darker side to this. The desire to inflict pain and the pleasure taken in witnessing it sometimes seems all too near the surface. In Chapter 8 Kate Maguire examines a subject most of us would rather not think about too much, in the light of her experience of working with the victims of torture. Not only have these people experienced indescribable pain (from which in many cases they continue to suffer) but they have been subjected to systematic attempts to rob them of all that makes them human. The stories are highly disturbing but Kate's reflections on what she has learnt from her patients, when she has been able to break down barriers of communication, contain valuable lessons for anybody trying to help pain patients who carry the scars of emotional trauma.

Much of the distress experienced by patients suffering in body mind or spirit is aggravated by their perception that doctors and other health professionals are failing to listen to what they are really trying to say: we may give the impression of listening but part of our minds are already occupied by other thoughts and we may only hear what we choose to hear. In Chapter 9 Andy Graydon contends that proper listening and effective communication require unfeigned sincerity, which he calls 'emotional sincerity'. When there are no barriers between us we can not only help our patients better but we can also learn and receive far more from them than we give them. He illustrates this by his accounts of conversations with Michelle, a woman dying of cancer who was able to accept her situation with love and joy, and to whom this chapter is dedicated.

It is well recognised that illnesses all have physical, psychological, emotional, social and spiritual dimensions, and that all of these components need to be addressed for a state of health to be achieved. This is explicitly recognised in the diagnosis and therapeutic management of alcoholism and addiction, and the well-known Twelve Steps of Alcoholics Anonymous have helped countless sufferers to come to terms with these aspects of their illness. In Chapter 10 Paul Martin and Paul Bibby describe a similar approach to incurable disease and intractable suffering.

The first meeting of the group was titled 'The inevitability of pain?'. People working in pain management programmes spend much of their time helping patients to come to terms with and accept the fact that their pain is not going to go away, that no one has a magic cure for it and that the constant search for relief is not only futile but gets in the way of progress to more realistic goals such as restoring activity and coping with depression. Pain therapists also need to learn to come to terms with their own relative impotence – something which is very difficult to acknowledge when they have perhaps entered the profession with unrealistic ambitions and expectations of what they could do for suffering humanity, but faced with desperate people who may regard them as their last hope have found themselves unable to help. But acceptance of this reality is not the same as therapeutic nihilism, must not involve shoulder-shrugging detachment, and can be turned into something positive. In the final chapter I pose some questions raised by the paradox of acknowledging our professional responsibility to relieve suffering and acceptance of our impotence, not so much in the hope of providing satisfactory answers, but more to illustrate the need for these meetings and this book.

(There remains the question as to whether there is some pain or suffering which is intractable, truly intolerable and completely *un*acceptable, which in turn raises the subjects of euthanasia and assisted suicide. The latter would of course have required a whole chapter to do it justice, and in view of the volume of existing literature and public debate on the issue it was decided with some reluctance – and retrospective regret – not to include such a chapter.)

REFERENCES

1   Bonica J. *The Management of Pain*. 2nd ed. Philadelphia: Lea & Febiger; 1990.
2   Notcutt, WG. The Tao of Pain. *Pain Reviews*. 1998; 5: 203–15.
3   Capra F. *Tao of Physics*. 4th ed. Boston: Shambhala, 1999.

FURTHER READING

The following suggestions are for further reading for the non-specialised or non-medical reader.

➤ Melzack R, Wall P. *The Challenge of Pain*. London: Penguin Books, 1996.
➤ Wall P. *Pain, the Science of Suffering*. London: Weidenfield and Nicholson; 1999.

About the editor

Peter Wemyss-Gorman was a consultant anaesthetist at the Princess Royal Hospital, Haywards Heath until his retirement in 2000. He established a pain clinic in the early 1970s at a time when this was a relatively new concept. The realisation that 'medical' interventions were frequently inadequate to relieve chronic pain and that much more was needed to help patients live with their suffering led to the establishment of the first multidisciplinary pain management programme in the south-east of England. But even this failed many people, and the consequent dissatisfaction and uncertainty of purpose, shared by many colleagues, led to the meetings which he has organised since retirement, and which have provided the material for this book.

Contributors

Michael Bavidge was a lecturer in philosophy at the Centre for Lifelong Learning, Newcastle University, and ran the adult education programme at the university for 10 years. He is the author of *Mad or Bad?* (Bristol: Classical Press; 1989) – a book on psychopaths and the law, and, with Ian Ground, *Can We Understand Animal Minds?* (Bristol Classical Press; 1994). He is chairman of the Philosophical Society of England, which aims to encourage ordinary people (i.e. people who are not in academic institutions) to involve themselves in the discussion of philosophical issues. He has been a regular contributor to the Pain Society Philosophy and Ethics Group.

Paul Bibby was a consultant pain nurse with the Sherwood Forest Hospitals NHS Foundation Trust until 2009 when he was appointed Clinical Director of Pain Management Solutions Ltd (a private sector provider to the NHS of community-based pain clinics); and an honorary research fellow at Sheffield-Hallam University. He began developing an interest in pain management as a result of his involvement and post-registration training in palliative care. In 1996 he was appointed as a nurse specialist in acute pain at Doncaster Royal Infirmary, where he set up inpatient pain services. During this time he became increasingly involved in assisting clinical teams in managing patients with drug and alcohol problems. In an attempt to learn more about this group of patients he investigated various schools of thought, including the Twelve Steps of Alcoholics Anonymous. His relevant publications include an article on existential pain in the *Nursing Standard* (Existential pain. *Nursing Standard*. 2003; **18**(10): 23) and a chapter on Alcoholism and addiction: the management of spiritual pain in the clinical environment, in the book *Beyond Pain* (Pat Schofield (ed). London: Whurr Publications; 2005).

Diana Brighouse was appointed consultant anaesthetist to the Southampton University Hospitals NHS Trust in 1990. Her interest in chronic pain management started as a registrar in Oxford, and she was fortunate to work both as registrar and senior registrar with Dr John Lloyd (who with Dr Samuel Lipton is regarded as one of the founding fathers of chronic pain management in the UK). The continuing development of the psychosocial model of pain management in Southampton led her to take a one-year course in counselling and psychotherapy in London. Some of the theoretical basis of the course resonated with theories of existential philosophy and non-verbal communication that had formed part of her Master's degree in comparative spirituality. These seemed relevant to the complex patients who were being referred to the pain clinic, where the boundaries between the science and art of medicine are becoming increasingly blurred. She went on to train as an integrative psychotherapist at Regents College London, during which time the pain clinic underwent major structural reorganisation, resulting in the majority of work becoming primary care-based, and invasive pain treatments being dramatically reduced. The patients attending for secondary care had frequently been given multiple diagnoses, or were under the care of more than one hospital specialist Many had a mental health diagnosis.

The multidisciplinary pain team agreed that patients requiring psychological therapies would not all be suitable for behavioural therapy, and Dr Brighouse started a clinic offering longer-term psychodynamic therapy. Her chapter is based on both theoretical models of care and on clinical experience drawn from this clinic (although it should be emphasised that clinical details do not relate to any single individual).

The Right Revd Michael Hare Duke was born India in 1925. He read Litterae Humaniores and Theology at Oxford and completed his ordination training at Westcott House, Cambridge. He was awarded an honorary DD at St Andrews in 1994. After parish ministry in London and Bury, he was appointed Bishop of St Andrews, Dunkeld and Dunblane in 1969, where he remained until retirement in 1994. He has been pastoral director of the Clinical Theology Association, chairman of the Scottish Association for Mental Health and chairman of Age Concern Scotland.

His books include: *The Caring Church* (1963), *First Aid in Counselling* (1968), *Understanding the Adolescent* (1969), *The Break of Glory* (1970), *Freud* (1972), *Good News* (1976), *Stories, Signs and Sacraments* (1982), *Praying for Peace* (1991), *Hearing the Stranger* (1994) and *One Foot in Heaven* (2001).

He continued to work as a hospital chaplain until at 82 he was officially declared as too old, much to his disgust! Until recently prevented by declining health, he had attended all the meetings of the Philosophy and Ethics Group since its inception and had become its 'resident' guide in matters theological.

The Revd Father Andy Graydon studied for the RC priesthood at Ushaw College, Co. Durham where his specialised subject was spiritual psychology. He was ordained in 1979 and began hospital chaplaincy in 1988 at the Montagu Hospital in Mexborough, South Yorkshire. He became involved with the pain management unit at the Montagu Hospital and joined the team, seeing people who seemed to be suffering from something deeper than physical or emotional pain. Working with groups and individuals, he developed forms of meditation, talking therapies and relaxation exercises. He has recently taken on the mental health chaplaincy in Rotherham and Doncaster.

Kate Maguire is a social anthropologist and psychotherapist who specialises in the dynamics of power and pain. She has worked extensively in the Middle East as an anthropologist during periods of conflict. As a psychotherapist informed by anthropology, she has worked with survivors of torture and extreme experiences both in the NHS and for Medecins Sans Frontieres. One of her many roles has been to head the Doctorate in Psychotherapy for the Metanoia Institute and Middlesex University. She is currently writing on the multidimensions of pain, its concepts, language and treatment across individuals and cultures and its relationship to personal and political power. She continues to lecture in the UK and abroad and has a special interest in qualitative research and the use of metaphor in therapy to communicate experiences of pain.

Paul Martin worked until retirement as a palliative care physician in Dundee and Ayrshire. He qualified in 1981 from the University of Manchester Medical School, UK and after general training pursued a career as a consultant anaesthetist. Reflection on what it means to be a doctor as well as a patient and the notions of care rather than cure led him to change career and train in palliative medicine. His main clinical interest is in achieving acceptance and resolution in the face of incurable disease.

Willy Notcutt is a consultant in anaesthesia and pain medicine in Great Yarmouth. He qualified in Birmingham in 1970, and specialised in anaesthesia after working as a flying doctor in Lesotho, and although he has remained an anaesthetist, his main interest has been in pain relief. Sadly the options for treatment were often limited and many patients were being left in severe unremitting pain. This led him to consider the possibility of cannabis (which he had first come across being used medicinally in the treatment of alcoholism whilst working at the University of the West Indies in Kingston, Jamaica) for pain relief. He has played a dominant role in the development of a prescribable extract of this drug.

He is currently director of pain relief services, the lead clinician for the back pain team and runs a research team. He is also an honorary senior lecturer at the University of East Anglia in Norwich and chairman of the Special Interest Group of the British Pain Society for Philosophy and Ethics.

Ian Yellowlees is currently a consultant in pain management in the Northumberland Healthcare NHS Trust having previously established a new multidisciplinary pain management service at the Borders General Hospital in Melrose, which became nationally recognised as a centre of excellence, and a new service for the management of acute and chronic back pain dropping the 'classical' pain management programme in favour of a more flexible approach using education modules.

Since moving to Northumberland he has been developing a new service structure separated entirely from secondary care and working mostly on the telephone. The introduction of electronic patient records has raised the possibility of 'virtual' clinics, with a service for remote areas such as the Western Isles.

CHAPTER 1

The Tao of Pain

Willy Notcutt

[The Tao of Pain was originally published in *Pain Reviews* in 1998[1] (*Pain Reviews* ceased publication in 2002). I decided to revisit it in light of changes in thinking in the hope that the material presented stimulates further reflection on the nature of pain and to move on from the simplistic views dating back to Descartes which continue to limit understanding.]

> Tao is a thing that is both invisible and intangible.
> Intangible and invisible, yet there are forms in it;
> Invisible and intangible, yet there is substance in it;
> Subtle and obscure, there is essence in it;
>
> *Tao Te Ching*, chapter 21[2]

INTRODUCTION

Pain is a universal experience and yet still remains poorly understood and often ineffectively managed. For physicians, some of the difficulties that we encounter may be the result of the fundamental principles of thought that govern our western medical science.

The International Association for the Study of Pain (IASP) defines pain in physical and psychological terms as:

> An unpleasant sensory and emotional experience associated with actual or potential tissue damage, or described in terms of such damage.

An alternative definition of pain can be derived by adapting the quotation from *Tao Te Ching* (the main Taoist text) at the start of this chapter:

> Pain is felt by all but it cannot be touched. It cannot be seen or directly measured, but its patterns can be recognised. Elusive and ill defined yet it has substance and specific characteristics.

This is a very different view but few would disagree with it. Taoism is half psychology and half philosophy. Some follow it as a religion although it does not have a central moral code. Instead its principles could simply be described as a *Way* (Tao), which, if applied properly, will serve its follower well.

This chapter draws heavily on the work of Fritjof Capra. In his seminal book, *The Tao of Physics*, he eloquently explores the broader aspects of physical science and its parallels within eastern mysticism.[3] To explore pain using this same approach and perspective may deepen our understanding of a complex and elusive subject thereby helping in our practical management of the patient.

HISTORICAL PERSPECTIVE

Throughout recorded history man has struggled to understand pain. In biblical times it was seen not only as a punishment for sins committed but also as the means of cleansing one's soul. Buddha in his First Noble Truth saw pain and suffering as being an inevitable part of life. As science replaced theology as the dominant explanation of the natural world, pain came to be seen as the largely unavoidable and untreatable side effect of disease and therapy. The introduction of general anaesthesia in the mid-19th century was a historical landmark in the relief of the anguish of surgery itself. However, little attention was given to post-operative or other pain problems which remained poorly managed.

Towards the close of the 20th century physicians accepted that pain itself was a legitimate and necessary target for their therapeutic activity. Cicely Saunders, the founder of the modern hospice movement in the UK, pioneered the control of the pain of cancer whilst others started to tackle the often more difficult and complex problems of the long-standing pain from many chronic diseases. Then clinicians turned their attention to the acute pain following surgery, injury and acute illness (some 150 years after the introduction of general anaesthesia!). Parallel to the increasing therapeutic activity, there has been an explosion of knowledge about the physiology, pathology, pharmacology, psychology and sociology of pain over the last 40 years. Now in the 21st century chronic pain is being recognised as a disease state in its own right. However, whilst some patients benefit, many do not and all pain management services have huge reservoirs of unmet need.

Chronic pain is very common, particularly as we get older. In the past the aches and pains of the degenerative changes that develop as our bodies age would be accepted as part of life and coped with accordingly. More recently there have been a number of epidemiological studies showing that the incidence of pain is more widespread than previously thought. Furthermore, patients' expectations nowadays are much higher and increasingly clinicians apply their skills to help patients control their pain as effectively as possible. Some excellent results are achieved both with analgesic practice and with surgery such as hip replacement. However, this is only the tip of an iceberg of patients with unmet needs for the control of symptoms resulting from irreversible physical and mental decline. Our abilities to provide help for such patients are often very limited.

The treatment of pain has come far in the last 40 years but is still burdened by the old Cartesian approach prevalent in much of Western medicine. This has led to us viewing pain as a target to be located with scanners, bombed with chemicals, stabbed at with steel or cauterised with ice or fire. Even some psychologists seem to attack the problems using their own weapons with similar vigour. Unfortunately, no single approach seems to deliver reliably the sort of results that we would like. We still seem to focus on attempting to achieve a cure as we would if treating a hernia, rather than obtaining a fuller understanding of the patient's problem. We may also be failing to recognise our own limitations in therapy.

Medical journals and conferences present the latest knowledge as if new weapons and targets are being found in a war against a vicious enemy. The various campaigners document the successes of their newfound technology and techniques. Pain teams have been recruited to lead the fight on the surgical battlefields and in multidisciplinary clinics.

However, in the headlong clinical rush to develop the relatively new specialty of pain medicine, it is reasonable to pause and reflect. Should we be tackling pain with the same aggressive approaches that are used for more tangible diseases such as cancer or infections? All too often we find ourselves 'blindly' lashing out at the perceived enemy, but failing totally to make contact. We lose our way and, what is more important, we may fail to help our patients.

I believe that we often fail to reflect on the nature and meaning of the pain of our patients as they present to us. Instead we focus almost exclusively on therapies and thereby neglect the deeper understanding of this phenomenon.

THE TAO OF PHYSICS

The Tao of Physics, written by Fritjof Capra, has been a classic exploration of the links between eastern mysticism (particularly Taoist thought) and modern fundamental physics.[3] At first sight, these two domains seem to be poles apart. However, Capra shows that there are parallels and connections between the two apparent opposites. He demonstrates and concludes that there is a single reality, but that it is being viewed from very different perspectives.

As we have developed our knowledge about pain and its treatment, we have fitted it (or constrained it) within our current western model of medicine. Even though we cannot explain so much of what we see clinically, we hold on to structures, systems, and concepts that have been laid down over the last 200 years.

Physicians specialising in the management of pain are commonly confronted with the problem of understanding its nature and the variability of the presentation, and the response to therapy and management. The 'Gate Theory' of pain has been a major advance in the unravelling of some of the processes involved. It provided a simple mechanistic method of explaining some neurophysiological processes, whilst also giving some insight into the relationship between pain and the organism itself. Unfortunately, many have seen the Gate Theory in terms of a wiring diagram, thereby missing the original objectives of its authors in explaining some fundamental principles of pain.[4] The Western medical mind struggles in accepting and understanding pain as its effects ripple outwards into the psychological and social dimensions of the individual.

Might other perspectives exist? An example is the Chinese system of medicine, developed over the last two millennia but scorned by the West until about 40 years ago. Acupuncture has now gained acceptance as an orthodox treatment, but the Eastern explanations, based on systems of meridians identified with visceral organs, are thought to have little basis in reality. However, we now know that the neural projections from somatic and visceral structures overlap almost completely within the central nervous system. The viscera are therefore neurally integrated with the skin and the musculo-skeletal system. We now accept that there is a complex and continual interaction between somatic and visceral systems. For example, women who have chronic low back pain may experience an increase associated with the menstrual cycle. Likewise, women with dysmenorrhoea may experience severe back pain. When confronted with a complex pain problem, Western medicine usually focuses on the somatic whilst barely acknowledging that there may be a significant visceral component or influence. Unfortunately access to the visceral nervous system for exploration, testing and therapy is very limited. However, the Eastern acupuncture approach combines both, and through the system of meridians, the viscera are mapped to the surface. The practitioner may then work to restore internal harmony through surface stimulation of visceral projections. Perhaps the Chinese were ahead of us with their linking of visceral and somatic nervous systems, in concept if not in physiologically accurate detail.

Interestingly both Western and Eastern approaches may be effective in both explanation and therapy. Here then, is a demonstration of a single reality (pain) being understood and treated in radically different ways according to different traditions and systems of medicine. Yet, at the neuro-physiological level, we can now see some ways of linking the explanations.

A DIFFERENT APPROACH

In his book *The Tao of Physics*, Capra presented six new paradigms of scientific thought, arising from his explorations in physics and in mysticism.[3] If these principles are truly fundamental and universal then they must be applicable to the subject of pain (and even to the whole of medicine). Capra himself touches on pain in his deliberations but does not explore it in depth. The purpose of this chapter is to look at pain using his paradigms in the hope that it will challenge some of our traditional concepts and ways of thinking and to help broaden our understanding of some of the complexities that we meet in our daily practice. I will present each of the six paradigms, outlining Capra's own definitions initially, and then develop the theme to apply to the subject of pain. I have cited quotations from the Taoist text, the *Tao Te Ching* (using two alternative translations), to provide further illustrative background and food for thought.

This presentation has some different perspectives on pain and my objective is to stimulate further thought, study and debate. However, this cannot be a definitive study for Capra's paradigms indicate that it is intrinsically impossible to provide one!

First paradigm

When you organise, you must of necessity use names and order.
But given that, you must also know where to leave off naming and structuring.

Tao Te Ching, chapter 32[5]

Knowledge of the structure does not predict function

Capra's first paradigm concerns the relationship between the part and the whole. In the mechanistic, classical, scientific paradigm, it was believed that for any complex system, the dynamics of the whole could be understood from knowledge of the parts. Therefore one broke the system down into pieces to find the fundamental building blocks and their laws of interaction. From there, one could explain the larger whole in terms of the properties of the parts.

However, Capra believed that it is not possible to understand fully the properties of the parts without knowledge of the dynamics of the whole. The parts cannot be well defined and they may show different properties depending on the context in which they are examined. Scientists from other disciplines have gradually realised that we have a universe that is more a network of relationships than one of fundamental building blocks. Thus we have a unity and a mutual relationship of all things and events. These are seen as interdependent and inseparable and as transitory patterns of the same ultimate reality. This type of approach has long been recognised by the proponents of gestalt psychology.

At medical school I was taught about pain by people who had taken the nervous system apart. I learnt of receptors in the skin, of different types of nerve fibre, of the structure of the spinal cord, of synapses, of tracts conveying signals to and from specific areas of the brain, and so on. Neurophysiology revolved around learning about the electrical activity of the nerve and the simple chemistry of its synapses. Thus I had been given the basic building blocks and their interactions. They taught me how a physical stimulus initiated a neural signal that was conveyed to the sensory cortex, how a motor impulse was in the opposite direction, how the release of endocrine hormones was finely regulated by negative feedback neural controls, etc. From this basic, physiological knowledge it was possible to understand the simplest alarm function of the painful stimulus.

This reductionist approach as the basis of much medical practice is very successful in the management of an acute illness where simple diagnosis leads to appropriate corrective therapy. However, for most health professionals, this is as far as it goes. It is difficult, for example, to go further and use this approach to predict the variability of the patient's response to acute or chronic pain, or understand the sensory alterations of 'wind up' or allodynia (experience of an innocuous stimulus – such as touch as painful) after acute injury. Unfortunately these phenomena are rarely recognised as important or, if noticed, are merely seen as inconveniences whilst undertaking the important therapy to treat and cure the patient of the underlying disease. Worse still, these factors are often not even noticed, especially by surgeons, who are themselves an important aetiological factor!

Variations in pain experience are seen elsewhere. The same neural channels convey stimuli that can be intensely pleasurable in one situation and extremely painful in another (e.g. loving sexual intercourse versus forced penetration). We often see one person who can largely ignore the pain of a specific pathology whilst another finds that it dominates his life. Many cultures have attitudes to painful events for which the individual will not express any pain. Amongst the Masai of Kenya, both ritual male circumcision of adolescent males and childbirth are expected to be experienced in silence without any acknowledgement of pain or requirement for therapy. A visit to a hospital in a different culture may show very different responses to pain by patients. Conversely, the neglect of pain management is very common and widespread.

In the mid-1970s a deeper understanding of the cellular mechanisms started to emerge based on the chemistry of the nervous system and the means by which neurons communicated. As a result the neurons are no longer seen as one-way conduits of a message. Intra-neural activity altering the way the signals are transmitted, inhibition, excitation, retrograde signalling across the synapse, and the chemical environment of the cell in the extra-cellular-fluid, have become all part of the new understanding of neural activity. In recent times there has been an explosion of interest in the role of glial cells in the functioning of the neuron and neural transmission. The neuro-chemical network becomes more complex the more we explore it. Therefore trying to explain or predict outcomes from this knowledge becomes even more impossible than before.

Dimensions as building blocks

Melzack wrote of the multidimensional nature of pain and the current IASP curriculum uses this terminology as do many others.[6] Therefore describing the basic elements or parts as dimensions rather than using the more traditionally based 'building blocks' is worth exploring. In principle, this is not new. The current wisdom is to describe pain as having sensory/discriminative, affective/evaluative and cognitive/behavioural components. However, this approach jumps from the older, mainly anatomical, approaches to one based strongly within psychological terms.

A dimensional approach to pain does not have quite the same apparent irreducibility as that of mass, length and time, or of a subatomic particle, but it remains fundamental in its own right. However, this approach allows the introduction of the important concept of complexity that is rarely considered in the understanding of pain. In the physical world we can only think of three spatial dimensions but mathematically the number is limitless. Some physicists currently find explanations for the universe in more than 10 dimensions, including ones that are 'wrapped up' (string theory, etc.). Most of this is unimaginable to our minds. However, by drawing some parallels with a multi-dimensional universe, we may get further insights into our pain world. I am suggesting this approach as a different approach and an idea for discussion but it should not be taken as literally as if these were the classical physical dimensions.

First dimension: neural architecture

The first dimension reflects the neural and glial network (three dimensional in a strictly physical sense). Previously we thought of pain being transmitted one way along 'wires' performing the simple task of raising an alarm. Descarte's classical picture of a boy with his foot too close to a fire is commonly used to demonstrate this concept. However, we know that the reality is a network of neurons forming a pathway in more than one direction and with lateral integration throughout. This is not just a bundle of cables; it is a three-dimensional structure with a specific architecture.

To this neural network of 100 billion neurons must now be added the glial network. Previously the glia were thought to be relatively inactive supporting structures (physical and immunological) for the nervous system. Now they are seen as having importance and probably essential involvement not only with normal neural transmission and modulation but also with pathological processes. Therefore a further layer of physical complexity is added to the neural architecture of the system.

Despite this apparent complexity, the analytical, structural, 'hardwired' approach works well in acute medicine where pain is seen as the alarm signal pointing to the site of a recent event. It rapidly starts to fail though as we try to understand the ramifications of pain as it persists. Frequently there is no obvious active pathology requiring the 'alarm' signal. Many patients go through prolonged, intensive, invasive and even dangerous investigations whilst the doctors try to elicit the exact cause of the chronic low abdominal pain or low back pain (as examples). Inconclusive results are common and explanations elusive.

New imaging techniques such as fMRI (functional magnetic resonance imaging) are now able to show specific areas of the brain which become more active under different pain states. It is very tempting to jump to the conclusion that these are 'pain centres' and link them up in some mechanical model forgetting that each area may reflect the activity of tens of millions of neurons. However, this is probably little more than looking through the casing of a desktop computer and seeing areas of general activity. It gives no information of what is happening at the microscopic level of the processor. Therefore whilst fMRI is providing information on the functioning of areas of the brain it is still a long way from providing an understanding of pain based on the way the areas of the brain are interacting.

It becomes clear that knowledge merely based on the anatomy of neural structures of the nervous system and the method of propagation of a nerve signal is wholly inadequate when trying to understand pain. From a look at the wiring diagram of a silicon chip it is not possible to explain why the words are appearing on my laptop as I type this chapter. Despite this, a visit to most textbooks will reveal illustrative wiring diagrams of the nervous system to show how the 'alarm bell' is rung but going no further in enabling the reader to gain a fuller understanding of what is really happening.

Second dimension: chemical

In the mid-1970s the endogenous opiates and their receptors were discovered and since then there has been an explosion in the understanding of the molecular chemistry of the neuron and associated cells. An increasing number of receptors and ligands that appear to be involved in pain have been found and the complexity of synaptic excitation and inhibition has grown. In the periphery, it was thought that each sensation had its own histologically defined nerve terminal that produced a response to a specific stimulus. Now the chemistry of the receptors themselves seems critical and currently 12 different types are recognised. Primary afferents code differentially for different stimuli types (heat, pressure, acid, etc.) and for intensity. Within the neuron itself the complexity of the chemistry is gradually being exposed both in the synaptic area and within the rest of the cytoplasm and the nucleus. Therefore it becomes very easy to try to define the fundamental building blocks of pain in terms of chemical locks, triggers and keys. However, this apparent simplicity vanishes when we realise that there are more than 250 chemicals identified as being associated with the pain system.

Furthermore, we now have to recognise the importance of the chemistry of the glial cells and the complexity seems to be steadily increasing. Therefore trying to understand and predict pain in chemical terms is not possible.

Third dimension: psychological and psychiatric

Over the last 40 years the exploration of the psychological dimension of pain has probably been as great as the physical. Whilst personality traits may influence pain, it is cognition that seems more important. It has certainly become a major target as can be seen with the rise of cognitive behavioural therapy over the last decade.

Depression and anxiety and their associated phenomena are very common but may not reach levels identifiable with psychiatric disease. Whilst a part of the pain process they may in themselves become as dominant factors as the pain itself. All psychiatric disease may have varied impacts on pain but as yet we have limited knowledge of the impacts (e.g. personality disorders, addiction, psychosis and organic brain disease).

The placebo effect is often treated with scorn and thought of as just a response of the patient to a dummy medication, whether in treatment or in research. The main psychological processes mediating placebo analgesia are those of conditioning and expectancy and have been studied in depth focusing particularly on the patient/clinician relationship.[7,8]

It is now realised to be a much more complex response and some say that it is one of the most powerful tools of pain management that we have. Conversely, the less studied nocebo effect may be equally powerful in rendering therapy ineffective.

Whilst these factors are essential components of pain they cannot be seen in isolation from other dimensions. Yet the use of the term 'psychogenic pain' is still common, implying as it does a singular cause and dimension, often reflecting the clinician's failure to cure with physical approaches ('It must be all in the mind.').

Fourth dimension: social

Social factors are an important extrinsic dimension. Whether it is acute or chronic pain that is being studied, the influence of such factors as bereavement, litigation, unemployment, family and friends, financial difficulties and culture on pain can be enormously powerful and complex. Commonly they are bundled with the intrinsic psychological factors and are clearly closely linked. The way in which culture, for example, may influence our response to pain is essentially a learned behaviour and so could arguably be placed in the third dimension.

Fifth dimension: temporal

Time is often spoken of as the fourth dimension of our physical world and has a linearity. The evolution of pain as a survival mechanism is the foundation of memory. From this emerged the phenomena of sensitisation, a protection against future harm. Past life experiences, such as physical abuse, are also now recognised as critically important in influencing the patient's current response to a noxious stimulus and maybe particularly important in the evolution of long-standing pain.

We commonly divide pain into three groups, namely acute, chronic and cancer related. Whilst the first by definition starts at time zero and resolves quickly, the second is defined by convention to start at three months (or six months) rather than with any specific event and the third has an onset and a potential finite end in death. The latter two might be better termed persistent or unresolved pain.

Time is a part of treatment when we consider pre-emptive and patient-controlled analgesia. There is a general recognition that the longer uncontrolled pain persists, the more resistant the pain becomes to treat. Therefore time is a critically important dimension of pain though rarely recognised as such.

Sixth dimension: genetic

The genetic dimension of pain is an emerging subject but its importance is barely understood. It seems intuitive that genes will be shown to have a significant role in the pain experience just as they are being shown to have in most other areas of physiology and pathology. Investigations of genetic influences upon nociception and pain have revealed genetic polymorphisms underlying specific pain phenotypes. Melzak identifies the 'Neuromatrix' of the brain as having a structure and function that is genetically determined.[6] Gender too has a bearing on the pain experience though this may also be through psychological or cultural mechanisms.[9,10]

Some of the differences that are seen in the response to pharmacological agents (effectiveness, side effects) are likely to reflect genetic variability. We already recognise this in the varied way patients respond to codeine. In the future, optimal pain control may be achievable through understanding of these molecular-genetic mechanisms, yielding individualised analgesic regimes.

Seventh dimension: unpleasantness

Fundamentally, pain is an unpleasant experience, otherwise it would lose much of its protective purpose. However, unpleasantness can also be a result of many other non-painful experiences (nausea, vertigo, vomiting, thirst, abnormal heart rhythms, abnormal sensations, etc.). It is difficult to define but we all recognise the concept. However, we may find it very difficult to fully empathise with the subject's experience. It has a quite different relationship to nociceptive stimulus intensity and may be influenced by various psychological factors. Therefore unpleasantness can be thought of as a further dimension of pain although many will place it within the dimension of psychology in the, 'affective/evaluative' bracket.

Unpleasantness has been described as primary or secondary.[11] Primary unpleasantness arising from an intense pain (or other) experience is easily understandable. It may also be a feature of nerve damage. Patients with post-herpetic neuralgia (pain after shingles) often give some of the most graphic descriptions. They may describe this in unusual terms ('rats crawling under the skin', 'block of wood'). The sensation and the hypersensitivity (allodynia) may be much worse for the patient than the actual pain intensity component.

Conversely we often meet patients who are needle phobic, who wince and grimace even with very little noxious stimulus. This is understandable for the patient who has a history of repeated and traumatic cannulation by a poorly skilled doctor and could be defined as secondary unpleasantness. For some though it appears to arise without preceding factors such as with other phobias. The experience of light touch when joined to the belief that it is a spider can produce extreme unpleasantness in an arachnophobe without any prior history of trauma, physical or psychological. Pain during a therapeutic massage may be a pure sensation like pressure and have a minimal unpleasantness component because there is no perceived threat.

Then there are those who get pleasure out of pain, whether in sport or in unusual sexual practices. Whilst the experience of pleasure is not the direct opposite of unpleasantness, I noted earlier that the same peripheral neural structures serving pleasure can be involved in generating pain (e.g. sex organs).

Eighth dimension: metaphysical

A metaphysical dimension to pain is an important dimension for many patients and clearly has been for millennia. Those who believe that there is no spiritual aspect to life, the universe, etc. will dismiss this dimension and place it within the realm of psychology or culture (third and fourth dimensions). For many patients a religious belief may provide some fundamental basis from which an understanding of pain can emerge in the context of disease, violence, torture, etc.

Conclusions

It is possible to argue for further dimensions and I considered including the immune system. Alternatively one might divide up one of the dimensions already described. However, the fifth paradigm shows that such descriptions are going to be approximations.

The importance of describing these eight dimensions lies in consideration of the implications. If we study the physical world we can easily understand the three-dimensional cube and also visualise it as a two-dimensional drawing. If we step up a physical dimension, we move to the hypercube which is impossible for all but a few to imagine. It can be modelled dynamically as a three-dimensional object with computer animation and as a two-dimensional graphic.[12] Moving beyond this becomes mathematically possible but visually unimaginable in any coherent way (except to those who explore fundamental physics possibly).

What emerges from this is a realisation that, like the universe, the dimensions of pain are well recognised. However, if we try to use them to produce and predict a functioning model of pain then even the minds of Einstein and Hawking would find it impossible. In pain as in physics, there is a huge chasm to bridge to link the basic elements to an accurate understanding of the way in which the whole system works.

The observation of the individual in pain has helped us gain a deeper understanding of the function of the various elements but it has not enabled us to predict the performance and the experience of the individual in any given circumstances. The specialist, who focuses just on neural pathways to explain pain and then treat his patient accordingly, will commonly fail to achieve lasting results. The whole history of neural ablation (neural 'wire-cutting') is a prime example of the limitations of this unidimensional approach to pain management. Yet many clinicians still base their therapy on single physical interventions targeting what they perceive are malfunctioning elements of the nervous system. Unfortunately results are often ambiguous and commonly of little long-term value.

Of course, pain processing is more than just 'wiring' as shown above. As the chemistry of the nervous system has been identified there is still a belief that if we can identify and list all the receptors and ligands at the synapses, then we will somehow have answers to the response of the nervous system when a noxious stimulus is applied. Then using this knowledge, we will know what chemicals to introduce to control the system. Those who focus on the psychology of pain can have similar 'mechanical' approaches looking for the specific technique which will resolve the problem.

The current IASP curriculum for trainees aims for an organised-structure approach to the subject of pain.[13] However, whilst all the elements are there that one is supposed to know, there is no attempt to show how it fits together. The trainee can be left with the box of pieces of a hugely complex jigsaw without a picture to guide him in assembly. Ultimately though, a knowledge of these structures does not predict the pain that a patient experiences.

Second paradigm

> Clay is moulded into a pot
> But it is the emptiness inside that makes it useful …
> … Therefore, existence is what we have
> But non-existence is what we use

Tao Te Ching, chapter 11[5]

Process is primary and determines structure

Capra's second paradigm emphasises the shift of thinking from terms of 'structure' to terms of 'processes'.[3] In the past it was considered that fundamental structures were acted on by forces and mechanisms, ultimately giving rise to processes. However, Capra believes that this is the wrong way round. It is the process that is primary and every structure that we observe is a manifestation of an underlying process. This paradigm complements the first one. Evolution is a prime example of the way in which the structure of the organism evolves according to how it functions in its environment.

When taught neurophysiology, I learned about nerve pathways, and viewed synapses as merely relay stations on the way from the periphery to the brain and back again. It was the functioning of that structural pathway that was important and defined. There was less concern about the function of the overall system. This was reinforced clinically by the neurologists who spent their time eliciting exotic physical signs to locate lesions deep within the nervous system. The resultant rigid taxonomy of disease marginalised those patients who did not fit, ejecting them into the lap of the psychiatrists.

Pain itself is now better understood in terms of the way in which the whole system functions rather than the pathway that neural signals travel. We know that it is the soup of chemicals that bathe a multitude of synapses that is all-important. These chemicals are released by both neurons and glia, thereby ensuring a dynamic electrochemical interaction of every neuron with its neighbours and not just with the targets of its neural projections. This complexity is made even greater when one starts to consider the role of the intra-neural transport of chemicals, the intracellular transmitters and the gene function within the nucleus in the generation of pain. Therefore the function of each neurone is not only dependent on all those surrounding it but also affects the function of all surrounding neurones, thereby forming a dynamic network.

Melzack and Wall described their 'Gate Theory' of pain in the mid-1960s and showed the principles by which the function of the neurons in the dorsal horn can be influenced thereby modifying the experience of pain.[14] Factors such as depression, boredom and anxiety could now be linked to alterations in spinal neural function, thereby altering the pain perceived. However, Wall never liked the theory as commonly expressed in textbooks. He saw that it would become a simplistic mechanism to explain the way in which the pain system worked. A visit to current textbooks commonly shows the wiring diagram with little in the way of explanation to aid understanding of the concept of pain.

Others have attempted to update the theory but it has remained a successful description of the overall neural processes involved in the dorsal horn of the spinal cord. For the clinician this is adequate. However, the basic scientist the theory is too general and therefore inadequate to quantify the various changes that neurons undergo after the onset of nociceptive stimulation.

The way the brain processes incoming information was described by Melzack in Neuromatrix Theory.[6] The concept of the iterative processing of signals principally between the thalamus, limbic system and sensory cortex shows how the brain generates the experience of pain individual to each person and each situation.

New papers on the physiology and pathology of pain bring new complexity and new difficulties in comprehending the integration of the various elements of the system in both health and disease. It is like a huge multi-dimensional spider's web of interactions. It can be recognised by all but mathematical definition is elusive. Adjust the tension in one strand of a normal spider's web and every other component alters its tension, and its relationship to its neighbours. Yet its structure is defined by its purpose. An example of this is the way in which wide dynamic range neurons in the dorsal horn, which are an important part of the nociceptive pathway, do not always sub-serve pain.

It is common to think of the nervous system as a static system with a fixed number of neurons that we steadily lose over our lifetimes. However, it is now well recognised that this is false. Under pathological circumstances such as long-standing pain, the nervous system can change substantially both in physical architecture (sprouting of new synapses, sympathetic baskets – 'malignant rewiring') and in neuronal and glial function. Alterations in the gene expression can occur leading to alterations in the quantities and types of neuropeptides produced; receptors may change or disappear; ion channels may change in number and location, etc. Reverberating circuits may induce permanent positive feedback loops causing up-regulation of systems. Thus the 'process' can not only change the physical functioning of various elements but also induce actual physico-chemical alterations in the architecture of the system. Pain not only generates changes but is also amplified by the changes. Worse still, in some chronic pain states, fMRI imaging has shown an increased loss of neurons in certain areas of the brain. As yet we do not know if this is an outcome or a cause of chronic pain (or even both).

When we think of structure, we usually only consider the physical. However, each person has a definable psychological and social structure and most pain physicians readily identify major changes in these areas as pain takes hold. It is common to see patients who have become miserable because of pain and not sleeping only to find themselves in a vicious spiral of depression, insomnia and pain. This can result in changes that range from the modest to the catastrophic or frankly bizarre. Too often, we experience patients with chronic pain and with grossly distorted lives. Unfortunately, it can be next to impossible to determine accurately the pre-morbid state.

When one superimposes psychological, social, environmental and spiritual dimensions onto the physical, the result is a 'structure' of increasing complexity. This is only understood in terms of a dynamic unitary network in which every element is functional and an integral part of the process. Palliative care physicians have long used the term 'total pain' to bind together and emphasise the oneness of these factors. Can any pain now be realistically considered in narrower terms?

The way in which the pain process restructures a person's whole life is often seen. A simple example will suffice. A man injures his back and loses his heavily physical job because he is off work. He gets depressed which aggravates the problem and causes friction within his family. He receives state benefits that are in excess of what he would have if merely unemployed. He sues for compensation. No one will now employ him with his record of back pain. He does not have the education or facility to retrain, and anyway, there is a shortage of manual jobs. The resultant state that develops is one that moves further and further away from the pre-morbid one, becoming increasingly resistant to treatment. The pain stays, physical function remains significantly impaired, the family becomes dysfunctional and the cost to the community increases. This is not a neural problem. It is a dynamic, complex situation where chaos theory probably rules and a physical, psychological and social catastrophe is generated. Our organisational and therapeutic resources are commonly inadequate to cope with these disasters.

These concepts have an important bearing on our clinical practice. The vigorous and effective early management of the process of pain is now believed to be not only beneficial to the patient but also critical to prevent the development of chronic pain. The corollary is that ineffective initial management of a patient and his pain can be an important part of the process that can have long-term physical, psychological and behavioural effects, thereby altering the function of the nervous system in ways that may become irreversible. The pain clinician might have a role that is more important in the controlling of the emergence of chronic pain than in the treatment of the resultant chaos once it is established.

Perhaps one of the most alarming phenomena seen by pain specialists is the way in which a complex regional pain syndrome can develop after an apparently minor injury. This is only understandable if seen as a pathological and persistent derivation of the 'wind up' process. What triggers this has yet to be determined but it is unlikely to be a single factor. A complex, psychophysical reaction of the whole system to the injury sustained is much more probable. In spite of much research no one is any clearer as to why this occurs.

Third paradigm

> What we must do is see the whole world as our 'self'.
>
> *Tao Te Ching*, chapter 13[5]

The observer is part of the whole system

The physicist Heisenberg incorporated the crucial role of the observer into quantum physics. He believed that we can never speak about nature without at the same time speaking about ourselves. There is no such thing as detached objective observation. Capra shows that in quantum physics, the observer and the observed reach a point where they can no longer be separated.[3] Similarly, mystics in meditation can arrive at a point where the distinction between self and non-self breaks down.

Every observer of pain interacts with the subject. Most people cannot watch a patient suffering severe pain without experiencing some empathy themselves. Behavioural studies in animals have demonstrated this latter point and fMRI studies in man confirm changes in localised brain activity. Furthermore these changes are more pronounced if there is a familial relationship between the observer and the sufferer.

Even if one is inactive, there are effects on the observed. Therefore, to stand by totally disinterested could aggravate the suffering of the patient by inducing a feeling of abandonment. Anyone conducting research into pain knows how the expectation, questioning, assessing and management of the patient during a clinical trial can significantly influence the evaluation of an analgesic technique.

When pain is long-standing, the relatives and acquaintances of a patient are initially observers. As time goes by they may quickly become deeply involved (for better or worse). At one end of a spectrum is the overprotective and over-supportive spouse who may even be gaining from the situation in some way. At the other end is the uncaring and frustrated spouse who is seeking greener pastures. Both may become a major component of the patient's problems, sometimes needing as much 'management' as the underlying pain itself.

Most of us who are involved in pain management will have experienced the situation of merely sitting and listening ('observing') to someone pouring out their heart about their pain and associated problems. Without any other significant therapeutic intervention or instruction we can find that the patient has actually benefited from this catharsis. The observer ('listener') has thus influenced the observed. Traditionally, doctors and other health workers have been taught 'never to get involved', 'never to show emotion', 'to remain detached and disinterested', etc. Clearly this teaching is nonsense, as all contact with a patient will have some effect, for good or for ill, or for both. It has been a long-held belief that the patients of the kind, gentle, listening doctor with a good bedside manner seem to do better. Some will even describe this as a 'gift of healing'. The corollary is that the 'bad' doctor, who is rude, rough, arrogant and fails to listen probably has an adverse effect on the patient. These positive and negative influences are seen as contextual effects and commonly described as the 'placebo' and 'nocebo' effects of the therapist on the patient and the outcome of therapy (*see* Implications for research on page 25).[7,8] Most pain specialists regularly see the casualties of previous medical practice, some cause casualties themselves.

There is a further aspect to consider. We cannot just think of the therapist as the 'observer'. Just as we affect the patient with his pain, the reverse must also be true. The patient is an observer of us and, by definition, must have some effect on us. This will then alter our further interactions and thus becomes an iterative process constantly shifting the relationship. When we consider the effect on us, we tend only to think of the negative side. Many believe that the continued exposure to the critically ill, the dying and those with chronic debilitating illness induces insensitivity, or worse, callousness. This is certainly true for some. Personal observation suggests that the most vulnerable to this effect are those doctors and nurses who have a mechanistic approach to their patients. Unfortunately, this approach is still a dominant factor in the training and practice of most Western doctors. Add to this the excessive workloads and the high levels of stress that many work under, and the result is the dehumanisation of patients. They quickly become identified only as 'diseases' and 'machines to be fixed'. Fortunately though, there have always been large numbers of doctors for whom the patient probably has the opposite effect, thereby bringing out the 'best' in such carers. The history of medicine is full of such examples and current-day medical practice is no exception.

There are more subtle changes that occur in all of us through repeated exposure to these patients. No one notices them, but they must be there. Commonly we observe the development of 'clinical experience' and equate it to a maturing wisdom. However, there are much deeper changes than mere medical skill. These affect our attitudes, emotions, enthusiasm, realism, etc. Sadly though this can again be a negative effect leaving professionals burnt out or indifferent. It is not uncommon to hear pain clinicians speak disparagingly of their patients and even state that all 'chronic pain patients are mad'.

Consequently, if we are continuously being subtly changed, then there must be a change in our own effect on the patients themselves. Therefore the relationship between observer and the observed is dynamic, two-way, complementary and ongoing but never static, easily defined or predictable.

Fourth paradigm

> Trying to explain it will only exhaust you.
> It is better to hold onto a paradox.

Tao Te Ching, chapter 5[5]

There are no fundamental equations

Capra's fourth paradigm concerns the foundations of knowledge.[3] The development of science over the last 500 years has been based on measurement. In physics, there has been a search for the fundamental equation, constant or principle upon which the whole understanding of the universe can be based. So far, each new scientific discovery or revolution has undermined or superseded older theories.

In cardiovascular, respiratory and renal physiology, the interrelations between pressure, flow, resistance, output, etc. are all easily described. Simple mathematical equations can be derived, computers programmed, monitors set and pumps turned on. The patient's life-support systems can then be managed along similar lines to flying a modern jet. Other physiological processes can be similarly harnessed.

Provided that the equations are not pushed beyond certain limits, they work reasonably well. In general, we study the parameters in zones of comparative stability which can be likened to the strange attractor concept from chaos theory. Once we go past certain limits the systems develop chaotic tendencies suggesting that the equations of chaos theory are probably more appropriate.

Pain is unlike most other physiological systems in being a subjective experience for which there is no exact definition, no hard measurements upon which to construct basic equations and no tidy theories to enable us to plan and predict the response to pain therapy. The visual analogue score (VAS) and numeric rating scale (NRS) are perhaps the closest that we have to measurement tools and are widely used in research. In reality, they are merely scores for an individual to rate his own personal pain experience. Whilst a blood sugar level of 5 has some concrete meaning across a population, it is difficult to interpret what a NRS of 5 really means to different people

It is still widely believed by many doctors and nurses that they can predict the amount of pain a patient will experience for a given situation. This is demonstrated by the rigidity of the prescribing of analgesics. Patients who express more pain than expected or who fail to have their pain adequately relieved by a specific analgesic dose are described as 'overreacting' or as having a 'functional' element to their pain. Little thought is given to the possibility that the initial predictions might be based on gross misconceptions. The advent of patient-controlled analgesia allowed a more liberal approach to the delivery of analgesics and has also released the doctor from the difficulty of prediction of pain for prescribing purposes. The patient analyses the 'data' concerning their own pain and operates a device to deliver more analgesia. However, the device, which may contain a small computer, merely regulates the dose and frequency of administration. It cannot be programmed in advanced to predict the correct amount of analgesic needed for pain control. Furthermore, a patient may use it to give some pain relief up to the point where side effects occur. Therefore, the dose administered is neither a direct nor an indirect measure of pain or the need for relief. Yet it is still widely used to assess the effectiveness of analgesics.

In the third paradigm we recognised the importance of the observer and the profound effect that he can have. However, we have no fundamental mathematical principles or facility for the measurement of this effect. Therefore, the prediction of the outcome of pain management relies essentially on experience, intuition and guesswork. We use an interconnecting network of models and theories to guide us as we try to find a more harmonious and comfortable state for the patient. In reality the individual determines the impact of the pain experience and his own requirement for its management.

The basic rules of mathematics which we use successfully elsewhere do not apply here. Applying the concepts of chaos theory is probably a more appropriate approach but naturally makes prediction of outcome an impossibility. Furthermore, applying conventional statistical methods as used in clinical trials for numerical data, in these circumstances becomes questionable. Each patient is an individual and as such only very broad principles can be applied.

Fifth paradigm

> She who knows that she does not know is the best off,
> He who pretends to know but doesn't is ill.
>
> *Tao Te Ching*, chapter 71[5]

All descriptions are approximations

For his fifth paradigm, Capra describes the shift from truth to approximate descriptions.[3] The older Cartesian paradigms were based on a belief of the certainty of scientific knowledge. However, in the new paradigm it is recognised that all scientific concepts and theories are approximation. Science can never give any complete definitive understanding as it always deals with limited, approximate descriptions of reality.

One of the biggest difficulties I routinely have to confront is the problem of providing patients with a realistic explanation for their chronic pain.

This is of course not exclusive to the specialty but is particularly frustrating for patients when there is no obvious pathology that can be linked to their experience.

Consider a common situation. A patient comes with back pain but does not have an easily defined prolapsed inter-vertebral disc or major structural abnormality. Therefore the mechanistic world of the orthopaedic or neurological surgeon, in which patients ideally have cause, effect and treatment clearly identifiable, has now become unclear. Quickly the patient is in the same situation having previously believed (or been told) that they had a 'disc' or a 'trapped nerve' by their GP.

It is well known that X-rays of the spine are poor indices of the causes of pain and loss of function. It is common to see patients with gross structural changes in their spines due to osteoarthritis and yet experiencing little or no discomfort. However, others, with minimal evidence of macroscopic radiological disease, are prostrate in agony. Despite this, doctors will readily leap to use the radiological abnormality to provide the patient with a complete explanation for their problem. The illogicalities are ignored or missed. Commonly patients are given wrong explanations which can have a variety of effects. When told that a 'disc has popped out' they believe that it can be 'popped back' in again. This is reinforced by clinicians who believe that they can do this despite their being no evidence for it (MRI scans). Then there is the acute localised pain in the back which is diagnosed as a 'trapped nerve', the understanding being that it can be 'released'. This is quite different from the true 'trapped' nerve of a prolapsed inter-vertebral disc. Sciatica is a widely used diagnosis, yet in truth is only a symptom of pain radiating down the back of the leg. I often see the 'diagnosis' applied to pains in other locations in the legs!

Other false diagnoses can have a greater impact. I often see patients who report that they have been told that their back is 'crumbling', usually associated either with degenerate discs or with osteoporotic collapse. This is not only completely untrue but leaves patients with the impression that their back is similar to a digestive biscuit and believing that a single movement might cause further deterioration. This can enhance catastrophising by the patient reinforcing immobility. Some patients see their MRI scans and the degenerate discs which appear black on the screen. The patient then picks up the idea that the discs themselves are actually dead or dying, enhancing their concern about their condition and future prospects.

The presence of a real structural abnormality may tempt the surgeon to offer surgery or the pain clinician to perform an injection. The combination of the patient's insistence on a cure combined with medical enthusiasm and blinkered vision has failed many. Pain relief clinics are littered with patients who have had multiple operations and procedures on their spine but who either have experienced no useful improvement or have been made worse.

The term 'the failed back' is widely used by doctors despite there being no such pathological condition. This implies a failure somehow on the part of the patient to improve. The fault is not the therapist's, who has done his best against intractable pathology and is thereby absolved of responsibility. It is interesting that we do not describe such patients as 'the back surgeon's failures', although this might be a more accurate term in most, if not all, circumstances. We rarely ask the question, 'Was the decision to operate correct?', preferring the opinion, 'It was worth giving him a chance'. Having seen patients who have had eight or nine operations on their backs for pain I have wondered when both surgeon and patient were going to realise the futility of the approach. How much the operations might contribute themselves to the ongoing pain is rarely considered. A belief often starts to grow that the patient's pain has a significant psychogenic elements. Next stop is a referral to the psychiatrist.

The Clinical Standards Advisory Group (CSAG) report on back pain in 1994[15] suggested that we stop focusing on diagnostic labels, except for the few patients who have clearly identifiable causes (e.g. vertebral compression fracture, prolapsed intervertebral disc, ankylosing spondylitis). The majority of patients can be grouped under broad headings such as 'simple back pain'. This shifts the focus from intensive, useless investigation to rapid, simple and potentially effective management using broadly based principles and an approach that is adapted to the individual's needs and responses. More recently, reviews of spinal surgery have cast significant doubt on the effectiveness of surgery for back pain (e.g. fusion). Even the simple concept of decompression of a disc compressing a nerve root may not be the optimal treatment. Pain clinicians too are not absolved here as most of their invasive treatments of spinal pain have a limited scientific basis and are not well substantiated by clinical trials.

We continue to use the term chronic pain but when exactly does the pain become 'chronic'? Is it at six months, three months, two weeks or is it at the point when the normal expected resolution of an acute event has not occurred? Is there a tipping point when suddenly the situation becomes irreversible or is there a steady accumulation of change towards a new position of stability, one in which pain is central. Therefore 'persistent pain' might be a more realistic description, placing the focus on a continuing process extending beyond an initial acute episode, rather than a static state that has been arrived at. There is a further problem with the word 'chronic'. In the UK this is often used as a description of quality not merely duration.

Most Western clinicians have been brought up in the rigours of diagnostic accuracy and classification that works well for much organic pathology. However, for pain, we have to accept the untidy and inexact world that is much closer to that which the psychologists inhabit. This is very uncomfortable for many pain clinicians, commonly coming from the realms of anaesthesia, a discipline that is very practical and mechanical in its approach. The medical education system prepares them poorly for uncertainties of pain management.

Sixth paradigm

Heaven's way is to nourish not harm

Tao Te Ching, chapter 81[5]

A leader who is advised to rely on the Tao
Does not enforce his will upon the world by military means
For such things are likely to rebound

Tao Te Ching, chapter 30[5]

Co-operation not dominance

Capra's final paradigm moves away from observation of nature and more towards advocacy.[3] He proposes a shift from an attitude of domination and control of nature to one of cooperation and non-violence.

The immune system, one of the body's protectors, can become overactive or work abnormally. There is sometimes a need to 'damp' it down and the use of steroids in rheumatoid arthritis is a simple example. However, if the immune system is damped down too far, the result can be rapidly catastrophic, as is sometimes seen with patients undergoing transplantation or intensive chemotherapy.

The pain system, which is integrated into the immune system, is similarly protective and in principle little different. In the acute situation it protects from further harm. In the recovery from injury it protects from excessive use of an injured part to allow healing. In arthritis it protects from excessive use of a damaged structure. For the patient with an osteoporotic spine and two collapsed vertebra, it shrieks out in protest under the mechanical load of a bag of shopping.

Total absence of pain can be profoundly damaging as seen with leprosy or Charcot's joints. The use of opiates or non-steroidal anti-inflammatory drugs (NSAIDs) are examples of how even therapy that reduces pain can have its downsides if pushed too far. Therefore there is a need to recognise that many painful situations have beneficial purposes, whilst at the same time we try to find ways to manage the excesses.

In the world of pain relief there has been a significant shift in attitudes to the approaches to treatment. In the 1970s and early 1980s, 'blocking' and destroying nerves and tissues was seen as the way to manage problem pains. Gradually, the emphasis changed, and the invasive, practical procedures have taken a second place to a broader bio-psycho-social approach to patients' problems. Nowadays many practitioners aim to minimise damage and to work with the systems that are malfunctioning, to try to restore some form of balance. Hence there is a move from inflicting violence on the nervous system to one of conservation, restoration and rehabilitation. At the psychological and social levels the invasive approaches have not been so marked, although there is still a potential for over-enthusiastic and possibly aggressive intervention.

Two important and linked problems hold back any changes away from the more aggressive, interventional approaches. First, the syllabuses for training doctors in pain relief still focus on the invasive aspects of treatment. Doctors like 'doing' things to patients, and when the largest group of doctors involved in pain management are anaesthetists, it is not surprising that regional anaesthetic techniques feature highly. Many consider pain management merely to be an extension of this. It is much easier to teach trainees how to do an epidural than to teach them why not to and how to convince the surgeon and the patient that it is inappropriate. It is also easier to talk about doing an injection than exploring sensitive issues in a past history that may include physical or sexual abuse.

A second problem lies once again in the language that we use (*see* the fifth paradigm on page 19). We still talk of 'pain killers' (modulators of neural transmission) and 'nerve blocks' (usually short-lived, pharmacological interruptions of neural transmission). Many years ago, I remember hearing two very experienced pain specialists describe themselves as 'needle jockeys'. For them, sharpened hollow steel was their main weapon of war and invasion their macho strategy. Many pain clinicians still work in this way believing that pain should primarily be treated by the insertion of thin metal probes into the body to deliver drugs, corrosive substances, heat, cold or electricity. The whole focus of a pain management service will depend on the enthusiasm of the practitioners for such techniques. In the introductory leaflet for patients for the pain management service of a prestigious university hospital, 80% of the information on treatment revolved around invasive physical techniques.

The disingenuous and prejudicial nature of our language and the labels we might use can be harmful. This is difficult when we still see pain as an enemy to be attacked on all fronts. Special interest groups operate within our professional pain societies and they attract enthusiasts who wish to develop a particular interest. These range from the physical to the psychological. However, there is a danger that such members will only view the treatment of pain in terms of the particular special interest. Hence one finishes up in the camps of either the 'needle jockeys' or the 'tea and sympathy brigade' (*sic*).

If pain clinicians have such divergent views, then we cannot expect other doctors to do better. How often are we still asked us to 'just cut the nerve ...' or 'inject the nerve with phenol ...' thereby to disconnect the patient from the pain. Their knowledge of the pathology of neural damage and all the consequent abnormal neural function is non-existent.

Patients and their families have the same conceptual problems. They too want to 'kill' the pain and expect that the latest medical weaponry will be targeted on their problem. Conditioned by the output of the popular media, they believe that anything less than total victory from such technology is unacceptable. They believe that in the 21st century we should be able not only to explain every problem but also to eliminate every unpleasantness. Yet the clinician who is a realist knows that compromise is essential in the management of pain, particularly when it is long established. The only achievable goal may be to try to help the patient remain on the right side of that fine line that divides the pain that can be managed from the pain that cannot.

There has been an explosion of psychological therapy for the management of pain. We perceive such methods to be benign but perhaps they too can be just as invasive and damaging as some physical procedures. Attacking pain behaviour and unlocking the past and its influence on the current problems may cause a significant upheaval for the patient, which when handled correctly may be therapeutic. What of those who cannot manage such therapy? Do we know anything about these casualties of psychological invasion and the long-term effects on their lives?

We have few long-term studies (years) of the benefits and side effects of any types of treatment of chronic pain. The variety of different multidisciplinary approaches reflects an older observation: 'When a lot of remedies are suggested, a disease can't be cured.'[16] There are now opinions that intensive psychologically based pain management programmes may not be as effective in the long term as their advocates claim. Therefore we might now consider that minimum psychological and social disturbance is as important as the minimal physical disturbance and invasion that we already consider to be necessary.

There is general agreement that the management of pain requires a cooperative and coordinated approach to assessment and treatment incorporating physical, psychological and social elements. The multidisciplinary team is considered to be the optimal way of delivering this and a common philosophy is essential for success. However, bringing in an anaesthetist merely as the 'hired gun' to perform an injection, or the physical therapist to do a manipulation, or the psychologist just to sort out the emotional problems, can easily distort or fragment an approach that is usually aiming less for a 'cure' and more for rehabilitation and restoration of harmony.

The big academic medical institutions should be providing such multidisciplinary teams but most other more locally based pain services have few staff and a very limited range of resources. The availability even of a psychologist may be minimal and some services just provide 'injection therapy'. However, many practitioners try to provide a more integrated bio-psycho-social approach and if this is applied early and appropriately, then it may be just as effective as the 'multidisciplinary' team. Is there evidence to the contrary?

Perhaps all pain specialists should be generalists and be able to manage most or all the various aspects of most new pain problems successfully. Some patients will require a more interdisciplinary approach whilst a few with highly complex (and generally long-lasting and intractable) problems may need more specialist resources. However, targeting the potentially treatable before they become untreatable is surely a more realistic goal for our everyday practice and training programmes.

The outcome of spending time listening and talking to a patient and finding that this has helped them to come to understand and cope with their problem is an eloquent demonstration of this paradigm, and a never-ending source of amazement. The emergence of fMRI as an experimental tool to explore pain has demonstrated significant changes within the brain as a result of non-invasive interventions.

Many years ago a colleague described pain clinicians thus: 'We rarely cure, we often help but we always listen' (R Atkinson, personal communication). The ear and the mouth may be the most effective tools for pain management that we have. This puts the much derided and so-called placebo effect of the therapist (another linguistic problem!) into a very different light. Perhaps the technophile mono-therapists could ease off a little and observe that there are other ways to manage pain that may be more effective and more realistic for the long term.

Maybe the approach of the conductor of a symphony orchestra is a useful analogy. Sometimes minor adjustments of instruments and modification of playing styles is required to turn a discordant noise into a more balanced and harmonious performance. Removing all the violins is not the solution. If we recognise that our individual 'treatments' rarely cure then our approach should be more about nudging the nervous system into a better balance. Sadly this concept can easily become 'Westernised' if we try to 'fine tune the machine' rather than trying to improve the playing style.

IMPLICATIONS FOR RESEARCH

Most research into the treatment of pain focuses on the basic sciences. Clinical research is almost exclusively on single elements of management viewed over short periods of time. Long-term studies are very scarce. The contents of the leading journal in the field, *Pain*, reveals very few papers comparing the outcomes of different treatment regimes and most concern acute pain only. This has changed little in 10 years.

Basic science research has given us an expanding insight into some of the mechanisms at work. However, different mechanisms for pain genesis probably exist within a single clinical diagnostic group. Furthermore, different patients with similar or identical diagnoses may need very different treatment strategies. The complexity of the pain state makes it essentially impossible to tease out single elements of physical or psychological pathology reliably for therapy without at the same time considering the many other aspects (first and second paradigms).

It is entirely possible that several elements of therapy need to interact to achieve significant improvements. Conversely, to leave out any element may lead to total failure. Therefore the study of single items of therapy (e.g. a specific 'nerve block') to try to obtain the answer, 'Does it work?' may be fundamentally flawed. Similarly, we recognise that 'dirty drugs' such as amitriptyline, which have a multitude of actions, are often more effective than highly specific agents such as the newer antidepressants. Morphine, another dirty drug, is still the gold standard with respect to opioid analgesics, rather than one of the newer synthetic analgesics.

There is a further problem. A therapy is not delivered in isolation from the therapist. The patient, the therapy and the therapist are a single dynamic process. It is often observed that the same treatment works differently in different hands. Therefore studying the therapy alone without the therapist is illogical and does not relate to the normal clinical situation. Many consider the therapist as an integral part of any therapeutic intervention and accept that this is one of the most powerful tools that we have in pain management. The logical extension of this is that when a patient does not improve, it may be more logical to change the therapist than the therapy!

The implications of the third paradigm for research are worse. Can we rely on either the patient or the observer to remain static for the duration of a study, particularly one that is long term? Can the observer be truly objective? Can we eliminate the positive or negative therapeutic effect of the practitioner from our studies?

The commonly used research tools work well when clinical problems are well defined such as diabetes, hypertension, etc. but can the same be said for pain? (fourth and fifth paradigms). Therefore using the same tools to study these different types of condition may be as sensible as using the same tools for both a hip replacement and an eye operation.

Perhaps the questions we ask are wrong. At what point do we measure outcome? Chronic pain is a continuum over a long period of time. Should we ever look at 'pain' as a single entity to be measured, as such, or should we approach from the direction of broad, functional assessments as we try to move the patient closer to a state of relative health (sixth paradigm)? It is therefore not surprising that no one has conclusively defined the place of epidural steroids, transcutaneous nerve stimulation and many other practical procedures in the management of pain of spinal origin. Yet most clinicians would recognise that a number of patients do improve after such treatment.

Many of the drugs used in the management of chronic pain are unlicensed for such use (e.g. amitriptyline). Sadly, the demands of regulators, academics and others, normally a long way from the front line of pain management, demand hard evidence before approving new therapies. If we have to wait for the results of gold standard, randomised, double-blind clinical trials before initiating any treatment then patients may be waiting a very long time for relief of their symptoms.

CONCLUSION

As the knowledge about the nervous system and about pain has grown, it has become progressively more difficult to understand it as a simple wiring diagram through which an alarm signal is transmitted. How we look at pain is going to depend whether we see it as a sensation, a symptom, an experience, a disease or a combination of all four.

The paradigms described by Capra[3] enable us to look at pain from a different perspective. At first sight the results of such an approach may seem nihilistic. However, much of the essence of Tao is in the art of *'wu wei'*, action through inaction. This does not mean, 'do nothing and wait for everything to get better'. What it really means is a practice of *minimal* action (particularly any that might be violent). To the outside world the sage appears to take no action – but in fact he is active long before others realise it (listening is a good example).

The reality is that pain presents us with huge challenges in basic understanding, assessment, diagnosis, management and sheer volume of need. Western medicine has provided us with some skills, medicines, technologies, etc. with which to take up the challenge of helping patients facing unremitting pain. However, the outcomes are very different from the results of such operations as joint replacement for the pain of osteoarthritis.

Understanding the pain is the first step, both for the therapist and for the patient, and it is critical to move beyond the 'Just kill the pain' type of concept. Capra's paradigms are an approach that may help this process thereby leading to management and research becoming more appropriate and realistic. As physicians, we ourselves are on a journey of continuing discovery. This chapter has been just such a personal exploration and I hope that it has encouraged others to stand back and consider just what it is that we are trying to achieve.

As therapists we sit at the junction between the past and the future with the opportunity of modifying the paths that patients will travel with their pains. Sometimes the way leads to cure. Commonly it leads to a modest improvement. For some, the road continues unchanged. Ultimately, like the physicist and the Taoist, we have to accept that pain is intangible, elusive and invisible and that patient and physician have to work to find the 'way' to work within this reality.

REFERENCES

1 Notcutt, WG. The Tao of Pain. *Pain Reviews.* 1998; **5**: 203–15.
2 Ch'u Ta Kao. *Tao Te Ching.* London: Unwin Paperbacks; 1985.
3 Capra F. *Tao of Physics.* 4th ed. Boston: Shambhala; 1999.
4 Wall P. On the relation of injury to pain. *Pain.* 1979; **6**: 253–64.
5 Mabry JR. *God as Nature sees God: A Christian reading of the Tao Te Ching.* Shaftesbury, UK: Element Books Ltd; 1994.
6 Melzack R. A multidimensional experience produced by multiple influences. evolution of the Neuromatrix Theory of Pain. *Pain Practice.* 2005; **5**: 285–94.
7 Richardson PH. Placebo effects in pain management. *Pain Reviews.* 1994; **1**: 15–32.
8 Finniss D. Placebo analgesia, nocebo hyperalgesia. *Pain Clinical Updates.* 2007; **15**: 1. Seattle: IASP Press.
9 Derbyshire S. Gender, pain, and the brain. *Pain Clinical Updates.* 2008; **16**: 3. Seattle: IASP Press.
10 Sufka K, Price D. Gate control theory reconsidered. *Brain and Mind.* 2002; **3**(2): 277–90.
11 Fields HL. Pain: An unpleasant topic. *Pain Supplement.* 1999; **6**: S61–9.
12 Wikipedia. *Hypercube.* http://en.wikipedia.org/wiki/hypercube.
13 Charlton JE (ed). *Core Curriculum for Professional Education in Pain.* Seattle: IASP Press; 2005.
14 Dickenson AH. Gate control theory of pain stands the test of time. *Br J Anaesth.* 2002. **88**(6): 755–7.
15 Clinical Standards Advisory Group. *Back Pain.* London: HMSO; 1994.
16 Chekhov A. *The Cherry Orchard* [play]. 1904.

FURTHER READING

➤ Aydede M, Güzeldere G. Some foundational problems in the scientific study of pain. *Philosophy of Science.* 2002; **69**: 1–17, Supplement for the proceedings of PSA 2000.
➤ Belzberg AJ. Commentary on Chapters 2–5. In: Cohen MJM, Campbell JN (eds). *Pain Treatment Centres at a Crossroads – A Practical and Conceptual Reappraisal.* Seattle: IASP Press; 1996. pp. 69–74.
➤ Berkley KJ. On the dorsal columns: translating basic research hypotheses to the clinic. *Pain.* 1997; **70**: 103–7.
➤ Capra F. *The Turning Point.* London: Flamingo; 1983.
➤ Clinical Standards Advisory Group. *Chronic Pain:* London: HMSO; 2000.
➤ Cohen SP. Management of low back pain. *British Medical Journal.* 2009; **338**: 100–6.
➤ Davies HTO, Crombie IK, Brown JH, *et al.* Diminishing returns or appropriate treatment strategy? – an analysis of short term outcomes after pain clinic treatment. *Pain.* 1997; **70**: 203–8.
➤ Giamberardino M. Visceral pain. *Pain Clinical Updates.* 2005; **13**: 6. Seattle: IASP Press.
➤ Goubert L, Craig K, Vervoort T. Facing others in pain: the effects of empathy. 2005. *Pain;* **118**: 285–8.
➤ Harstall C, Ospina M, How prevalent is chronic pain? *Pain Clinical Updates.* 2003; **11**: 2. Seattle: IASP Press.
➤ Kim H, Dionne R. Genetics, pain, and analgesia. *Pain Clinical Updates.* 2005; **13**: 3. Seattle: IASP Press.

➤ Lippe PM. Pain medicine: a conceptual and operational construct. In: Cohen MJM, Campbell JN (eds). *Pain Treatment Centres at a Crossroads – A Practical and Conceptual Reappraisal*. Seattle: IASP Press; 1996. pp. 307–14.

➤ Lainacraft G, Molloy AR, Cousins MJ. Peripheral nerve blockade and chronic pain management. *Pain Reviews*. 1997; 4(2): 122–47.

➤ Lennox JC. *God's Undertaker*. Oxford: Lion Hudson; 2007. Chapter 3, Reduction, reduction, reduction … pp. 52–6.

➤ Loeser JD. The future: will pain be abolished or just pain specialists? *Pain Clinical Updates*. 2000; **8**: 6. Seattle: IASP Press.

➤ Long DM. The development of the comprehensive pain treatment program at John Hopkins. In: Cohen MJM, Campbell JN (eds). *Pain Treatment Centres at a Crossroads – A Practical and Conceptual Reappraisal*. Seattle: IASP Press; 1996. pp. 3–24.

➤ Maruta T, Malinchoc M, Offord P, *et al.* Status of patients with chronic pain 13 years after treatment in a pain management centre. *Pain*. 1998; **74**: 199–204.

➤ May A. Chronic pain may change the structure of the brain. *Pain*. 2008; **137**: 7–15.

➤ Melzack R. From The Gate to the Neuromatrix. *Pain Supplement*. 1999; **6**: S121–6.

➤ Notcutt WG, Austin J. The acute pain team or the pain management service? *The Pain Clinic*. 1995; 8(2): 167–74.

➤ Price DD. Psychological and neural mechanisms of the affective dimension of pain. *Science*. 2000; **288**: 1769–72.

➤ Symreng I, Fishman S. Anxiety and pain. *Pain Clinical Updates*. 2004; **12**: 7. Seattle: IASP Press.

➤ Wager T. Placebo-induced changes in fMRI in the anticipation and experience of pain. *Science*. 2004; **303**: 1162–7.

➤ Wörz R. Pain in depression – depression in pain. *Pain Clinical Updates*. 2003; **11**: 5. Seattle: IASP Press.

ACKNOWLEDGEMENTS

I would like especially to thank the colleagues with whom I work, the participants at the British Pain Society's Philosophy and Ethics meetings, Bill McRae and Minha Rajput and many others for all providing me with a 'sounding board' for my ideas (crazy and otherwise) and stimulating new ones. Finally, I acknowledge the wisdom of Patrick Wall and his encouragement after reading an early draft.

CHAPTER 2

Suffering and choice

Michael Bavidge

Increasing patient choice has become a major theme in planning and improving health services. There are, however, problems about choice in relation to suffering and the experience of dying. Suffering and death seem to stand in direct opposition to freedom. Though our attitudes deeply affect the way we experience suffering and death, they are not activities. We undergo them. Suffering makes us dependent on others; to a greater or lesser extent we lose our autonomy; our power to act independently is lessened. Suffering undermines our ability to think clearly and act effectively; the dysfunctionality of suffering emerges in lack of choice. There are, of course, other inhibitors of freedom. Poverty and other forms of social deprivation seriously diminish our capacity to choose – but in an external way. Suffering undermines us from the inside. The suffering person has not got that ease and space in which we normally exercise choice. Suffering affects us at our core.

The threat that suffering poses to our viability as people is a challenge to healthcare strategies that place increasing emphasis on patient choice. Autonomy, freedom of choice and informed consent are part of the package of notions that go with consumerism and contract. If suffering seriously undermines patient independence and freedom of choice, the suspicion grows that the relationship between patient and carer cannot be modelled on the relationship between consumer and provider. In cases of minor medical interventions consumerism may capture the sort of relationship we want to have with the health service. But there is a gear change as soon as illness becomes a serious threat to health or suffering threatens to undermine our integrity as people. People who are seriously ill or suffering cannot act like consumers. Consumerism does not take sufficiently into account the intimacy and urgency of the relationship between carers and patients.

On the other hand – and here is the dilemma – loss of control and the curtailing of freedom are a major part of the experience of suffering and, consequently, any therapeutic regime must aim to increase patient control.

Despite the destructive impact of suffering on the range of patient choice we can at least reduce the apparent incompatibility by realising that there are different sorts of choice. Not all choices have the same structure; they do not all make the same demands on those who choose or those who react and respond to the choices; the roles that people are required to adopt in these transactions are not always the same. It may be that for those who are seriously ill one sort of choice loses its significance while another grows in importance. Not all choices are consumer choices.

TYPES OF CHOICE

Choosing a washing machine is a good example of consumer choice. The shopper knows roughly what she wants; she informs herself what models are available at what prices; she is competent enough to organise the finances and complete the various chores that are required to buy the item she has chosen.

Consumer choice in general presupposes:

➤ an array of well-defined goods
➤ a reasonably stable field of choice
➤ a consumer who is adequately informed
➤ who knows her own mind
➤ who has the necessary executive competence to satisfy her preferences.

But we make other sorts of choices which do not have these characteristics. We choose to get married, to enter onto a career path, to join a political party. These choices realise personal commitments. We think of our lives as having a trajectory over which we exercise at least some control. We think of ourselves as having an open-ended future which, whatever difficulties lie ahead, offers opportunities for a worthwhile life and self-fulfilment.

A choice of commitment in general presupposes:

➤ a set of ambitions or hopes which, though they can be characterised in general terms, are largely unspecified
➤ an open-ended and changing field of choice
➤ a person who has a reasonably realistic view of themselves and of the world they live in
➤ who looks to the future with a degree of hope and expectation
➤ who has the resources to maintain a course of action.

If we compare these lists we can see significant differences in all these elements of choice. A choice of commitment does not involve specific objects of choice as consumer choice does. We do not choose our spouses from the array on the shelf. The groom is asked, 'Do you take this woman to be your lawful wedded wife?'. The question does not mean 'Is *this* the woman you have chosen from all the available ones. Are you sure? Wouldn't you perhaps prefer this one?'. It means, 'Are you really committed to marrying this woman?'.

The field of choice determines what the person takes to be the available lines of action open to them. Our choices are shaped by what is socially available. We can only choose from what is on offer or what is being proposed. When we choose we take the initiative, but we are also responding to initiatives coming from elsewhere. In this respect choice is like consent. The *Oxford English Dictionary* defines 'consent' as 'voluntary agreement or acquiescence in what another proposes or desires'. Given the reactive nature of consent it is curious that in medical ethics it is tied so tightly into autonomy. It is a weak idea of autonomy that is spelt out in terms of giving or withholding consent to what others propose. The power to give or withhold consent may be an important element in autonomy – in the way voting in a general election is an important part of democratic life – but, if it is all that is available, it may well constitute a spurious alternative to autonomy – as voting once every five years may be an alternative to, rather than the core of, democracy.

So choice, like consent, presupposes a socially specified field of choice. But an important difference between consumer choice and commitment is that consumer choice requires relative stability in fields of choice. You cannot make a sensible consumer choice if when you get the goods home they turn out to be already worthless. You cannot make sensible consumer decisions when the annual inflation rate is 200%. Commitment choice, on the other hand, involves signing up whatever the future holds – for richer, for poorer, in sickness and in health. Commitment choices are open-ended and unconditional in a way that consumer choices are not. This open-endedness is inherent in the commitment. It is not something reluctantly acknowledged because, for example, marriages or careers last for decades and things are bound to change. Commitment choices mark the beginning of journeys that cannot be mapped out in advance.

Another point of comparison is the sorts of knowledge that are required to make good choices. The consumer needs information. She has to be well-informed. The term 'informed' enshrined in the phrase 'informed consent' has taken on a central and legally determined role in medical ethics. The importation of the word 'informed' into the clinic is not innocent or insignificant. We have come to talk about *informed* consent, not well-advised, or well-supported or sympathetically encouraged consent. This usage fits in with the way the word 'information' is used and with the way we have been told to think of ourselves living in the 'Information Society'. But the phrase 'The Information Society' is an oxymoron: we can all access the same information without forming a society. That is rather the point of information. It is knowledge cut free from its origins, from the individuals and the community that are responsible for it; it is stored, lost and found, bought and sold, manipulated and spun.

However, the choices we face in cases of serious ill-health require a much more personally engaged sort of knowledge than is captured by the word 'information'. What makes these choices difficult is not lack of information but poor understanding of ourselves and of the aims that we can sustain as our situation changes. This sort of understanding can only achieved through the sorts of conversations in which patients 'are able to express themselves clearly about *the things that matter to them*'. These conversations, which Eric Cassell believes are essential, can be difficult and time-consuming, but 'legalism, bureaucratic requirements, and formal consent forms are not an adequate substitute for such discussions'.[1]

There is an interesting contrast between the rhetoric of informed consent and the language of the hospice movement. Palliative care aims to transform the *experience* of dying; it is in the cognitive business, which is why the acknowledgement of death and candour with patients is central to its mission; but it does not aim to produce the best *informed* dying people.

Finally the consumer and the commitment maker require different sorts of competence. The ideal consumer has pretty clear objectives and she buys a product fit for purpose. She sees herself as a player, as counting, as having rights. She sees herself as entitled to good service and fair trade. The maker of commitments focuses not on contractual rights but on more general values. She is not in the business of pursuing particular objectives but of giving a shape and direction to her life. What she requires are not managerial or administrative skills but personal qualities that enable her to maintain some sort of positive orientation to the future. What she relies on are not her legal rights but her own inner resources and trust in the people on whom she depends.

SUFFERING

Bearing this distinction in mind we can see how maximising patient choice remains a viable objective even in cases of serious suffering. Loss of control is a contributing factor to the suffering that patients experience but, just for that reason, it is important to support patients in regaining control over the trajectory of their lives.

Suffering and pain are often used interchangeably or in tandem. It may well be that the most familiar cases of suffering are those that are caused by, or accompanied by, pain. Some pain may be so overwhelming that it is inconceivable that anyone could experience it without suffering. But there are differences between them which help to explain why suffering is an obstacle to choice and also demands an increase in choice.

We can be in pain and not suffer. The injured rugby player may be in pain and yet be exulting in victory. Equally, we can suffer and not be in pain. Psychiatrists see patients who are suffering severe distress and yet are not in pain. Sometimes suffering is so palpable that we refer to it as 'mental pain' as if it were a sensation. But it is not a sensation: it is not localised in the way pain is, nor does it begin and end in the way pains do. Pains have causes but not reasons. Our attitudes and thoughts do, of course, affect our experience of pain. But if we get burnt, the burn is a sufficient explanation of our pain. We do not normally have much use for the question, 'Why, having been burnt, are you in pain?' Suffering, on the other hand, has both causes and reasons. The death of a child will cause the mother to suffer. But it is not the death in itself without reference to the mother's thoughts and feelings that produces suffering. The death does not cause suffering more or less independently of how she takes it. There are reasons why we suffer and those reasons are integral to our suffering.

Suffering is a cognitively richer state than pain. We do not need to know much to be hurt by a flame. In this respect suffering is more like an emotion than a sensation. To love or hate someone, we have to know, or think we know, something about them. However, there is an important difference between emotions and suffering. Most emotions have objects. Fear and love are directed at the feared or loved person or thing. We hate or fear something or somebody. But there is no object of suffering. There are special cases of emotion that are also objectless – nameless dread, generalised anxiety or, to give a positive example, the oceanic feeling that we may feel listening to music. In these cases we ourselves play the role of an object. These states of mind are self-orientated; they have a reflexive structure.

Similarly, suffering has a quasi-object – our own vulnerability as persons. Suffering is a protracted, deeply unpleasant experience. It is the helpless distress we experience when we are overcome by the unbearable and the unavoidable. It is what we experience when we are faced with something dreadful – death, hopeless illness, loneliness, abandonment – that threatens to dismantle what we take to be the core of our personalities. It realises itself in despair, depression and anxiety.

Suffering affects the whole person and is a function of our sense of ourselves. The reasons we give when we try to explain suffering relate events to ourselves. We all feel very sorry about the death of a child and are upset by it. But the mother, with her aching love and unqualified commitment to the child, suffers. This is not to say that the reasons for suffering are selfish – the mother is not suffering because she has been made sad. But it means that they are self-orientated. She is suffering because her beloved child has died.

The cognitive richness and the reflective nature of suffering explain why it undermines our competence as persons. A searing toothache can immobilise us, but we are immediately restored to normal functioning if the pain can be alleviated. There is no such simple intervention to resolve suffering. It can only be alleviated by altering attitudes and feelings, by reorientating ourselves in the social world and by regaining control of the shape of our lives.

It is, consequently, to be expected that those who suffer are more likely to see their predicament in terms of commitment choices rather than consumer choices. 'Here I am – suffering. What is to become of me? What am I to do to make my life liveable again?' What appears to the non-sufferer to be a consumer choice becomes in the experience of the sufferer a commitment choice.

A consultant may explain to a patient diagnosed with prostate cancer the nature of the disease and advise him about various treatments. The patient is asked to choose which course of treatment he wants. NHS Choices tells us that according to the 2005 British Social Attitudes survey, 65% of patients want a choice of treatment.[2] No doubt most people would prefer to have a choice rather than have a particular treatment imposed upon them without consultation. Still what the choice of treatment means to the patient is likely to be quite different from the choice as it presents itself to the doctor. There is a danger that there is little meeting of minds between them because for the doctor the problem is an objective one of calculating the line of action most likely to produce the best result. But the patient cannot escape seeing the problem in terms of 'What am I going to do?' or 'How can I envisage living through these experiences?'. This is a general feature of choice for the suffering. Consumer choices are transformed into commitment choices.

So if we want to improve the lot of the sufferer we must try to maximise his opportunities for making commitment choices. It may be that without pain relief this is not a realistic possibility. All the attention and energy of the sufferer is taken up by his pain. Pain relief is necessary but it is not sufficient. He has to relearn hope; and rediscover the assurance that, however bad his situation, there are things worth striving for. He must be able to feel that, though his life may seem to be severely restricted, he still has a say in the shape his life is taking, even if, *especially* if, it is drawing to a close.

Achieving these aims involves modifying virtually every aspect of health provision. We need health professionals who acknowledge suffering, therapies that address the suffering patient, not just the disease or the symptoms of suffering, and institutions that provide an environment in which the reality of suffering is not denied.

Hospices are such institutions. The hospice movement started because Cicely Saunders realised that people need a place to die. Hospitals were not keen even to admit that their patients died. Death meant failure. So new institutions were needed that were committed to palliative care rather than cure. If hospitals found it difficult to admit that their patients die, they found it even more difficult to admit that their patients suffer.

Hospice literature is marked by frankness about death and pain management. As Ann Richardson expresses it: 'Still in the 21st century in the UK people die in avoidable pain and distress. In hospices multi-disciplinary teams strive to offer freedom from pain, dignity, peace and calm at the end of life.'[3] The word 'distress' is used in hospice literature rather than the word 'suffering'. This is not an accident – 'distress' acknowledges personal misery, but it sounds more episodic and more responsive to intervention than 'suffering'. As death is seen as failure by medical practitioners who are focused on cure, suffering is seen as failure by the hospice which is focused on making death a positive experience. There can be a 'good death', but there cannot be good distress or good suffering.

Palliative care that addresses the patient as a person, not just as a case, requires a language in which suffering can be expressed and responded to – not of course just a vocabulary, but a language that people can inhabit, underpinned by relationships that make communication possible and supported in an environment which does not force the sufferer into silence. The recognition of the need to allow suffering a voice underlies the hospice movement and the various forms of self-help groups that have sprung up to met the deficiencies of institutional healthcare. Sandra Clarke, one of the founders of the US program No One Dies Alone, puts it simply: 'The two things people fear the most about dying are being in pain and being alone.'[4]

MEANINGLESS SUFFERING

One of the main obstacles to controlling and therefore alleviating suffering is its meaninglessness. A central function of religious belief has been to give meaning to suffering. In Christianity, value is attributed to human suffering through its relationship to redemption and the suffering of Christ. But 'the problem of suffering' has become a growing source of embarrassment to traditional theology.

The term, 'theodicy', constructed out of the Greek words for God and justice, was introduced by *Leibniz*. In 1710, he published a work entitled *Essays of Theodicy on the Goodness of God, the Liberty of Man and the Origin of Evil*. In it he attacked Pierre Bayle who had claimed in his *Dictionary* that the *goodness* and *omnipotence of God* are incompatible with human suffering. Leibniz notoriously went for broke and established the compatibility of God's goodness and suffering by proving that, as he put it, 'this universe must be in reality better than every other possible universe'.[5] Voltaire poured scorn on his optimistic conclusions in *Candide*.

A spiritual account of suffering that avoids the offensive rationalisation that Voltaire detected at the heart of theodicy can be found in the reflections of Emmanuel Levinas. In his deep and subtle meditation entitled 'Useless Suffering', in which suffering plays a fundamental but paradoxical moral role, he wrote that the suffering of others 'solicits me and calls me … my own experience of suffering, whose constitutional or congenital uselessness can take on a meaning, the only one of which suffering is capable, in becoming the suffering for the suffering … of someone else'. 'It is this attention to the suffering of the other that ... can be raised to the level of supreme ethical principle ...'[6] but which 'cannot give itself out as an example, or be narrated in an edifying discourse'.[7]

This is not a moral theory that a practical social thinker like Aristotle or David Hume or Jeremy Bentham could advocate. It is, in a non-pejorative sense, a moral fantasy. But perhaps it is either this heroic response or nothing for someone who, like Levinas, was so aware of the fate of his fellow Jews, for whom, under Nazism, suffering had become the dominant mode of existence.

There are more down-to-earth attempts to make sense of suffering. Sometimes suffering is represented as the inevitable price of achievement – the 'no gain without pain' school. Some robust pedagogues no doubt think that there can be no education or discipline without suffering. It is hard to suppress a cynical thought about the recommendation of suffering on these sorts of ground: some experiences are so dreadful that they can only be borne if they are thought to be wonderful. Just as some actions are so wicked that they can only be undertaken for the highest motives. Surely there are less destructive and dangerous ways of cutting through trivia to the essentials of life? Suffering is not a positive experience even if by various stratagems we manage to draw benefit from it.

Retributive theories of punishment have found a function in suffering as a secular form of atonement. But we are no longer comfortable with the thought that suffering should be inflicted, even on criminals. Capital and corporal punishment have been abolished. We imprison people instead. Punishment is meant to consist of the removal of freedom and nothing more. Convicts are not expected to like prison, but neither are they expected to suffer there. Though we have to wonder why, despite a general fall in the suicide rate in the UK, there were 90 self-inflicted deaths in prisons in 2007.[8]

None of these religious, moral or social attempts to give some sort of function to suffering appear plausible or even decent nowadays. The uselessness of suffering may be part of the despair that we feel when we are in its grip. But there are dangers in thinking that suffering has a meaning. If you think suffering has a redemptive value you may even come to believe, as the Inquisitors did, that you have a duty to inflict it.

People of more theoretical inclination may find consolation in the thought that pain has evolutionary advantages. It warns us of damage or illness, helps to identify and locate the source of problems and discourages self-harming behaviour. Not all pains can claim such usefulness but it is a plausible story that our liability to pain has this sort of function. Suffering, on the other hand, seems essentially dysfunctional. It looks as if suffering is, in evolutionary terms, the incidental price we pay for knowing so much and becoming so refined and sensitive.

Failure to find a convincing theological or secular rationale for suffering may not be such a tragedy after all. The problem of suffering is not a puzzle. It is not a form of intellectual perplexity in which we do not quite know what to say. It does not take the form of a search for a convincing story to tell *about* suffering; it is the search for an authentic voice to speak *out of* it.

Maybe suffering cannot be given any function, earthly or transcendent, but it remains the thing we wish to avoid most. Enhancing patient control is an important part of any attempt to decrease suffering. The control needed will never be acquired through a set of consumer choices, but neither does it consist only in what is going on inside the patient's head. We want to control our lives as we experience them. The realities of our lives with which we are concerned here – suffering and the experience of dying – are shaped by our attitudes. Regaining control over those attitudes is regaining control over our lives. It is not a matter of despairing of changing the realities and settling instead for changing internal attitudes. Seeing choice in this light involves rejecting the dualism of inner and outer and the equally suspect dichotomy between physical realities and mental subjectivities. Eric Cassell's recommendation is relevant here: 'making objective and conceptually separating the thing that seems to be the source of the suffering can help lift its burden from the patient. This is important because to objectify is to provide for joint ownership and sharing of the situation.'[9] The patient is not alone. Of course, 'it must be absolutely understood that decisions regarding such courses of action are to be made by the patient. The patient, using the knowledge of the doctor, must decide what goals (not what treatment) meet his or her best interests or purposes – *no one else can know that*' (emphasis in original).[10] The triangulation that Cassell maps of the patient's predicament objectively described, his perceptions and apprehensions and the concern and care of others represents the best structure within which choices can be made – choices that are patient-centred, informed by professional advice and supported by carers, family and friends.

REFERENCES

1 Cassell, EJ. *The Nature of Suffering and the Goals of Medicine*. Oxford: Oxford University Press; 1991. p. 242.
2 www.nhs.uk/choices/Pages/Aboutpatientchoice.aspx
3 Richardson A. *Life in a Hospice*. Oxford: Radcliffe Publishing; 2007. p. x.
4 www.latimes.com/features/health/la-he-dyingalone4jun04,1,3632379.story
5 Leibniz GW. *Theodicy: Abridgement of the Argument Reduced to Syllogistic Form*. Available at: www.class.uidaho.edu/mickelsen/texts/Leibniz%20-%20Theodicy.htm
6 Levinas E. Useless suffering. In: Levinas E. *Entre Nous*. London: The Athlone Press; 1998, p. 94.
7 *Ibid*. p. 99.

8 National Institute for Mental Health in England. *National Suicide Prevention Strategy for England: annual report on progress, 2007.*

9 Cassell, EJ. *The Nature of Suffering and the Goals of Medicine.* 2nd ed. Oxford: Oxford University Press; 2004. p. 287.

10 *Ibid.* p. 283.

CHAPTER 3

The questions of pain

Michael Hare Duke

Any serious encounter with the experience of pain raises three interlinked questions demanding examination in separate categories. The first and most immediate concern is bound to be the clinical issue of its source and how it can be treated 'Why does my stomach hurt? What treatment does it require to take away the pain?' Before this can be effectively addressed a second more fundamental issue needs to be tackled as to why so unpleasant an experience is incorporated into the existence of all sentient beings. When anaesthetics were first discovered they were treated with suspicion by the medical profession. Because pain seemed an inescapable part of life, it was assumed to be an integral part of the given order of nature. Charles Meigs (1792–1869), Professor of Obstetrics at Jefferson Medical College, described the use of anaesthetics in surgery as 'a questionable attempt to abrogate one of the general conditions of man'. When this philosophical point of view governed clinical judgement the result could be disastrous. Sir Robert Peel, founder of the British Police Force and leading politician of the early 19th century died in 1850 as the result of a riding accident in Hyde Park in which he broke his collarbone, several ribs and a leg. Although chloroform was known he was not offered any pain relief and the bones could not be reset because of the agony that this would entail. He died after three days of excruciating pain, denied the right of any relief either by his surgeons' fear that they might kill their distinguished patient or by the controlling assumption that pain should not be opposed. The latter must also have been the attitude of the British army surgeons in the Crimean War when they treated the wounded and dying in the same way.

The third question that pain poses is the spiritual one; in what way does a person grow through his or her suffering? Perhaps the Crimean Army surgeons would have argued that the soldier who could go through the agony of an amputation without analgesics would be a more intrepid combatant. A similar approach to pain informed the educational values of the Greek City State of Sparta from the sixth to the fourth centuries BC. The ruling oligarchy believed that it was necessary for them to hold down as their serfs the indigenous Helot population that they had defeated. This required a tough regime of training. The exemplary story was told of a boy who concealed a fox beneath his clothing without giving any hint of pain as it gnawed at his intestines in order to disguise its presence.

Yet this was an attitude alien to most of the ancient world who would have concurred with the adage '*Divinum est sedare dolorem*' ('it is godlike to alleviate suffering').

Meanwhile the great world faiths, Judaism, Christianity and Islam have understood pain to have originated as a divine punishment for human disobedience. The myth took various forms: with St Augustine, humanity's deliberate rebellion had brought pain in the Garden of Eden; for Irenaeus pain was part of the incompleteness of creation but even so its possibility left the Creator as the author of potential suffering in apparent contradiction to his universal love. A coherent theodicy has to wrestle with the paradox that God was declared to be both Almighty Love and the Author of Ills Unlimited. This was summed up in a play in verse by Archibald Macleish based on the Book of Job, called *J.B.*, which won him the Pulitzer Prize in 1959. This propounded the theological dilemma in the quatrain:[1]

> I heard upon his dry dung heap
> That man cry out who could not sleep
> 'If God is God, he is not good
> If God is good, he is not God.'

As in the Book of Job, there is no rational answer; only a bullying response from 'God' ridiculing Job for daring to ask such a question.

This leaves medicine with the question of a moral understanding of anaesthesia: is it against the will of God? Does it deny the individual an opportunity of development when pain might have proved a method of character-building? Similarly if society uses pain as a form of social control, are those who alleviate it allies of the delinquents? At its least a significant level of pain can be a necessary early warning system of danger where a lesion is either invisible or inaudible. In the case of leprosy where the disease has destroyed all feeling, the patient is at risk of serious wounding by cuts or burns of which he or she is unaware. Therefore even from a physical point of view there is not a universal imperative to alleviate all pain and morality adds the dilemma of the double effect, where procedures for pain relief may pose a risk of shortening the patient's life. A value judgement has to be made as to whether the unalleviated suffering outweighs the gain from a period added to a patient's life. Into this will enter the further religious question as to what all concerned believe about life after death.

The Book of Job reached the conclusion that, 'Man is born to trouble as the sparks fly upwards' (Job 3:17); although the meaning of the original Hebrew is not entirely clear. Modern translations replace 'sparks' with 'birds' or 'eagles', but the sense remains that human life is inevitably fraught with discomfort. Pain in its universality takes us back to the ultimate question of responsibility. This has best been answered in story form rather than by logical argument. Christianity gives the account of Christ's Passion and sees the answer for each individual Christian to equate suffering with a personal vocation to follow the Way of the Cross. In the Gospel of Mark Jesus says, 'If any want to become my followers let them deny themselves and take up their cross and follow me' (Mark 8:34). Matthew and Luke include the same injunction. In his Letter to the Colossians Paul turns the idea round: 'It makes me happy to be suffering for you now, and in my own body to make up all the hardships that still have to be undergone by Christ for the sake of his body, the Church.' As the Early Church had to brace itself to cope with persecution it looked to the story of the Passion of Christ to give its own sufferings a meaning.

Taking another route, the poet Elizabeth Barrett Browning uses a myth to justify pain showing destructiveness redeemed as the source of music drawn from pan pipes:[2]

What was he doing, the great god Pan,
Down in the reeds by the river?
Spreading ruin and scattering ban,
Splashing and paddling with hoofs of a goat,
And breaking the golden lilies afloat
With the dragon-fly on the river.

He tore out a reed, the great god Pan,
From the deep cool bed of the river:
The limpid water turbidly ran,
And the broken lilies a-dying lay,
And the dragon-fly had fled away,
Ere he brought it out of the river.

High on the shore sat the great god Pan,
While turbidly flowed the river;
And hacked and hewed as a great god can,
With his hard bleak steel at the patient reed,
Till there was not a sign of the leaf indeed
To prove it fresh from the river.

He cut it short, did the great god Pan,
(How tall it stood in the river!)
Then drew the pith, like the heart of a man,
Steadily from the outside ring,
And notched the poor dry empty thing
In holes, as he sat by the river.'

This is the way,' laughed the great god Pan,
(Laughed while he sat by the river)
'The only way, since gods began
To make sweet music, they could succeed.'
Then, dropping his mouth to a hole in the reed,
He blew in power by the river.

Sweet, sweet, sweet, O Pan!
Piercing sweet by the river!
Blinding sweet, O great god Pan!
The sun on the hill forgot to die,
And the lilies revived, and the dragon-fly
Came back to dream on the river.

Yet half a beast is the great god Pan,
To laugh as he sits by the river,
Making a poet out of a man:
The true gods sigh for the cost and pain –
For the reed which grows nevermore again
As a reed with the reeds in the river.

Here the story is the product of the poet's imagination; it offers a metaphor for understanding the challenge of suffering, to see a way of coming to terms rather than resenting it. For Christian believers the Crucifixion claims to be history conveying a theological truth, not a parable to illuminate a problem.

With the growing number of old people in the make-up of the population, how they can relate to the physical and mental pain of old age is increasingly important.

This is an area for collaboration between medical and religious professionals in order to avoid bitterness and recrimination, a battle over resources in the NHS and a false expectation that if one group or another tried harder the situation would improve.

There is no clear or easy answer to the questions that pain presents. To manage the demanding situation lies within ourselves, our trust in one another and the confidence that we bring to our living and dying. Nevertheless the human spirit continues to look for a story that will help individuals find a coherent pattern in their suffering. This is evidenced by the popularity of a recent novel called *The Shack* by William Paul Young.[3] It starts with the horrifying account of a young girl's murder while on holiday with her family. Through a complicated sequel we follow her father as he retraces that holiday journey and confronts a fictionalised version of 'God' drawn from the Trinity but with the Father portrayed as a black woman, Jesus as a companionable human being and the Holy Spirit as a kind of etherealised Tinker Bell. Since Young appears to have had some training for the priesthood the theological analogies, though startling, carry plausibility. The publishers claim that the book has the potential for making a comparable impact to Bunyan's *Pilgrim's Progress*. Once again it seems there is a need for an interpretative story which will help a generation make sense of the violence and tragedy that feature so much in its experience, something that will restore confidence in the justice of Creation and of the Creator behind it.

REFERENCES

1 Macleish A. *J.B. J.B. A Play in Verse*. Boston: Houghton Mifflin; 1958.
2 Barret Browning E. In: Quiller-Couch A (ed). *The Oxford Book of English Verse, 1250–1918*. 2nd ed. Oxford: Oxford University Press; 1939. pp. 812–13.
3 Young WP. *The Shack*. Newbury Park, CA: Windblown Media; 2007.

CHAPTER 4

'Bundling with big pharma': ethics and the drug industry

Willy Notcutt

INTRODUCTION

It is a reality that most of the development of new drugs is undertaken by the pharmaceutical industry. However, many criticise doctors when they become involved with the industry and look upon them as being somehow tainted and therefore unable to maintain independence. Yet pharmaceutical and other medical industries need doctors to help with research, development and subsequent introduction of new medicines and therapies into practice. Doctors need new drugs and other treatments to improve the effectiveness of their practice. It is difficult to find people who have the necessary clinical experience but who also have the spare time and independence to work with feet in both camps, so to speak. Therefore to survive such a symbiotic relationship and avoid being sucked into the world of commerce a doctor may have to steer a difficult course.

There is much debate on this issue but little in the way of sensible, realistic or practical solutions. Therefore if there is no obvious answer, studying and identifying the ethical issues may be a useful way forward even if it only informs doctors about the potential pitfalls and problems that might arise.

BUNDLING

In times past when houses were small and travel was difficult especially in rural areas, a young man having visited his betrothed might find himself needing to stay overnight at her home. To give the young couple some privacy, the parents might allow them to share the same bed. However, maintaining chasteness was a problem and so the concept of bundling emerged. The basic idea was simple – how to avoid full sexual intercourse.

There were many different methods of bundling. In the Middle Ages a bundling board (a body-length piece of wood) was secured upright between the lovers but this was easy to get over. Sewing the boy and/or the girl into a 'bundling bag', a linen sheet that would bind, confine and conceal the legs and torso became a common technique. Boys with Houdini-like talents might be bound right up to the neck in a bag, with their hands tied behind their backs! Occasionally, the more liberal parents might allow above-the-waist nudity, since it could hardly result in pregnancy.

I originally presented on the topic of our relationships with the pharmaceutical industry to a meeting of the Philosophy and Ethics Special Interest Group of the British Pain Society. I wanted to explore the problems of working alongside the pharmaceutical industry in developing a major 'new' pharmaceutical whilst at the same remaining independent and 'distanced' from commercial issues. In this chapter I will be reflecting on my own experiences with the pharmaceutical industry although the principles remain the same for other medical technologies.

The objective of this personal essay is to explore the ethical questions, dilemmas and pitfalls that I have encountered whilst working in the development of medicinal cannabis. The study of a drug that has a long history and a 'criminal record' has been a unique journey in itself. Some other issues have been drawn from the wider experiences of myself and others, and not just in connection with the pharmaceutical industry.

However, in these reflections, I am not targeting criticism at any specific company or individuals I have been working with. It will be for readers to decide how successful the 'Bundling' was in my own involvement with industry.

BACKGROUND

Cannabis has a therapeutic history of some 5000 years. Research into the medicinal benefits started in India in the early 1800s. A physician, William O'Shaughnessy, brought this knowledge to the UK in 1842 and research into its use for managing pain continued to the end of the century. However, it was superseded by morphine and aspirin both of which had been purified and provided predictable analgesia, particularly in acute pain. The difficulty in providing a standardised preparation of cannabis was a big problem.

In the 1930s political and commercial pressures lead to the rise of 'Reefer Madness' campaigns to eliminate hemp as a cash crop in the US. Ultimately cannabis was condemned as a drug of addiction with no medical use. The World Health Organization sought its worldwide ban and by 1971 it became no longer possible to prescribe cannabis as medicine in the UK.

Fortunately research into the basic science continued and eventually the mechanisms of action started to emerge. The endogenous cannabinoid system was discovered in the late 1980s and suddenly it was realised that there was a whole unexplored physiological system here and an explosion of basic research followed.

Sadly this was not matched an explosion of clinical research. In contrast, morphine had become a proven therapy for pain long before the discovery of the endogenous opioid system. Anaesthetics continue to be used since their discovery in 1846 despite a lack of knowledge about their mode of action!

There were four main reasons for this. First, it had previously been decided that cannabis had no therapeutic potential, perhaps more by those who were non-clinicians. Secondly, the stigma of cannabis being a drug of addiction remained. Thirdly, there was no standardised preparation that would fulfil regulatory requirements. Fourthly, smoking cannabis was recognised as an unacceptable mode of delivery clinically, and alternatives would need to be developed.

By the mid-1990s a number of people with multiple sclerosis and other chronic diseases were 'coming out' about their use of cannabis for their symptoms. They wanted the liberalisation of the laws on cannabis so that they could gain legitimate relief from their pain. The anecdotal evidence was strong but not adequate to change the status of the drug. Inevitably this got mixed in with the call by others for changes in the law on the recreational use.

My interest in cannabis as a potential agent for relieving pain started in the early 1990s and was derived from knowledge of its historical use. I was seeing many patients who were getting inadequate analgesia from the drugs and other techniques available. Surprisingly, the synthetic cannabinoid Nabilone was available. It had been licensed in the 1980s for the treatment of nausea and vomiting secondary to chemotherapy. Whilst it was effective, it commonly caused dysphoria thereby limiting its use. The advent of the H_2 serotonin reuptake antagonists provided a range of new anti-emetics that were much more effective, so Nabilone became an orphan drug. Although it was not licensed for such use, I started to use it for treating intractable pain problems. About two-thirds of patients got some benefit but half of these found the side effects excessive. All patients who had also used cannabis in the past found it preferable to Nabilone.

To this day only two radically new types of drug have emerged for use in chronic pain over the last 40 years, Gabapentin/Pregabalin and ketamine. This is unlike most other areas of medicine such as hypertension, asthma and cancer, etc. where a large range of medicines have emerged over the last 20 years. In pain management, a wide range of drugs are used which are not conventionally identified as analgesics and are unlicensed for such use.

As I studied the history and anecdotal evidence, I came to believe that it was necessary to explore the use of cannabis primarily for chronic pain. Previous studies in the 1970s had focused on comparing it with conventional analgesics for acute pain. Using better methods of investigation we might be able to establish whether there was clinical evidence for what patients were telling us. The evidence from the basic science was very supportive and therefore we had an obligation to investigate cannabis fully and properly, or, alternatively, close the book on the matter.

Two main problems remained: first, the lack of a standardised extract of pharmaceutical quality and, secondly, the lack of a non-smoked, convenient delivery system. Overcoming these two hurdles would allow the development of high-quality research programmes to investigate the medicinal claims. Reviews of the literature had suggested that it was probably a safe medicine. No deaths directly due to the drug had been recorded and the dependency potential was thought to be low. The possibility of an association with the development of psychosis was recognised but at that stage unclear. Furthermore the whole issue was entangled with the ongoing debate on the recreational use.

In 1998 GW Pharmaceuticals was established to produce plant-based extracts of cannabis to be used initially in clinical research with the possibility of medicines emerging. Clinical research started in 2000 and an extract now known as Sativex emerged as a first product. Based on research carried out in the UK Sativex was licensed for clinical use in Canada in 2005. It became prescribable as an unlicensed drug on a named patient basis for compassionate use in the UK in 2006 gaining its full licence in 2010.

ABOVE THE PARAPET AND AVOIDING HAVING MY HEAD BLOWN OFF

In 1993 I decided to put my head above the parapet and start discussing in public the possible use of cannabis as a medicine. This started as a letter to the Guardian newspaper which put me in contact with the Alliance for Cannabis Therapeutics (ACT). The ACT was run by Claire Hodges who was a point of contact for those using cannabis medicinally and those wishing to find out more about the subject, particularly journalists.

Claire and I realised that we needed a set of rules to govern our contacts with the media. The first was to state clearly the separation of the recreational from the medicinal uses in any interview. I would cite an equivalent situation with diamorphine (heroin), which is widely used as an analgesic by doctors in the UK. In medical circles, no one discusses the recreational and the medicinal use of this drug at the same time.

In separating the two issues, I have always refused to discuss in public any issues around the recreational use nor have I ever given my own opinions on the legalisation of recreational cannabis (or any other drugs). To have done so would have compromised my goal of restoring cannabis for important medical uses. This stance proved successful and gradually we observed the media recognising the separation too. This led to me being able to refuse to participate in situations (e.g. live discussions) where the medicinal use was being tacked on to a discussion of recreational issues, sometimes, I believed, just to sanitise the debate.

I also realised the need to avoid 'pot humour' in general. There is a considerable culture surrounding the recreational use and inevitably I have had to know and understand the issues here, whilst pursuing my own course. However, it was essential to present a clean image and avoid comments that reflected the other side. Even words are important. I use the terms 'cannabis' not 'marijuana/weed/grass', etc. and 'cannabis cigarette' not 'joint/spliff', etc. wherever possible. This has been particularly important when speaking to transatlantic audiences.

DOCTORS WORKING WITH THE INDUSTRY

There are many factors that drive the doctor to become involved with pharmaceutical companies. Perhaps at the top comes intellectual curiosity and exploration at the cutting edge of medical science. The potential benefit to patients also comes high on the list. For many doctors there is a frustration at not being able to resolve clinical problems especially if basic science is clearly showing that there may be a way. The clamour for newer and newer cancer treatments is a classic example here.

The subject of money always rears its 'ugly head' and may come in several forms. Research grants from industry may be the chief source of funding for both basic and clinical research departments. The balance between conducting high-quality research and not biting the hand that feeds it may be a difficult one (to be explored below – *see* page 54). Sometimes research comes with an expensive piece of equipment which, if left behind after the project is finished, is a big carrot. Whilst funding may be an invaluable source of revenue for a department sometimes it goes into the pocket of the chief or principal investigator. Therefore, ensuring transparency of funding arrangements is essential.

The clinician or scientist who is involved in significant advances may now have the problem of fame to deal with. Whether it is the media or invitations to speak at international conferences in exotic locations, the ethical tensions are there. Having been flown to Whistler in Canada a few years ago to participate in a two-day meeting, I was able to stay over for a few days skiing afterwards (this latter part being financed by myself).

THE PHARMACEUTICAL COMPANY

Pharmaceutical companies are not in the business of science for academic interest, nor in philanthropy. The driver is to achieve success for the company and profit for the shareholders. This principle applies at all levels. Therefore anyone who is working on drug development risks being thus tainted and may even become a pariah to the rest of his colleagues.

At most stages of a drug's development, companies seek the advice of experienced professionals to ensure they are going in the right direction. When the development of a new drug may cost several hundred million pounds, the wisdom from clinical practitioners is of great value. Over the years I have been invited to a number of 'advisory boards' for a variety of companies and drugs. The fees paid are generally much less than paid in other non-medical industries compared with the potential value to the company. Seeing a selection of the data obtained from research informs participants and may influence their prescribing practice. Commonly they are already enthusiasts for the drug's development, and may be able to see the new drug's exclusive niche market.

As time has gone by, my personal interest and experience in cannabinoids has been recognised by a number of companies that have then sought my advice. Having worked closely with GW Pharmaceuticals in the development of its own drugs, I have had the problem of trying to ensure that I did not reveal any commercially sensitive information not already in the public domain (and vice versa). Difficult as it can sometimes be, I have not knowingly breached confidentiality in this area.

For most doctors the interaction with the pharmaceutical industry is at the level of the sales representative whose one objective is to promote sales of their product. They are commonly highly educated (some have PhDs) and are well trained in their job. Added to the information on the drug being promoted are the offers of pens and other low-cost items, food to accompany any technical presentations, help with expenses to attend conferences and in the past, even more. In recent times this has come under significant regulation. In recent times their codes of conduct have become more rigorous under the watchful eye of the Association of the British Pharmaceutical Industry.

MEDIA TRAINING: FIRE-PROOFING AND GAGGING

In 2004 it was anticipated that the cannabis drug that I had been helping to study would obtain its licence and go to market. As someone who had significant experience in the use of the drug, it would be likely that I would be invited to speak not only to doctors but also to the press. I had already been doing this for 10 years. However, the company that planned to market the drug decided that it might be beneficial for me to improve the quality of the messages I might give and, more importantly, to ensure I did not get tripped up by a combative interviewer. I therefore underwent some training in managing a variety of interview situations and in how to deal effectively with awkward questions. Having the skills to remain in reasonable control has certainly been useful on occasions and enabled me to say what I wanted to say. Most importantly it has enabled me to avoid such questions as, 'And finally doctor, tell me, have you ever smoked cannabis?'!

Fire-proofing has been useful to me and, by extension, to the pharmaceutical companies I have been involved with. It has also been useful to some of my medical colleagues when they have needed advice on handling the media. However, I do not think it has ever compromised the messages that I have sought to deliver. Rather, I hope it has enabled me to get them across. The company that undertook my training also teaches politicians and businessmen how to avoid trouble with the media.

I was asked to speak at a conference in Santa Barbara, California entitled 'Patients Out of Time' in 2007. This conference was to focus on the medical uses of cannabis (marijuana) and I believed was therefore within my self-imposed rules on public speaking (*see* Above the parapet on page 50). About three months beforehand I was asked not to go by GW Pharmaceuticals. I was informed that a theme of the meeting was lobbying for the liberalisation of marijuana laws so that patients could either grow their own or obtain supplies from an unregulated market. I had always seen this approach to the provision of cannabis as inappropriate for the administration of a medicine. I was also informed that GW Pharmaceuticals was involved in sensitive negotiations with the US government to embark on research there. It was felt that these could be compromised if one of the leading clinical researchers in the UK showed up at the Santa Barbara meeting. I had to ask myself whether I was being restricted in speaking on the subject for commercial reasons. It was the first time that this had happened. I resolved the issue by considering that the greater good might be served by my declining the invitation. Getting high-quality research underway with standardised, non-smoked cannabis medicines was the higher priority that should not be hindered, particularly by my attendance at an event that was itself unlikely to achieve significant outcomes.

CONDUCTING THE RESEARCH

Studying cannabis as a medicine brought a range of unusual problems not seen in most other studies. The initial target group was patients with multiple sclerosis (MS) suffering with spasticity and/or pain, and all had intractable problems uncontrolled with conventional medicines. MS is a disease presenting with a complex set of symptoms and many sufferers were frail. It was necessary sometimes to reject the worst-case patients on the basis that they would not prove satisfactory patients for the studies. There was, however, great temptation to bend trial protocols to enable as many patients as possible to participate and try the new medicine. These were desperate patients trying to find any relief they could from very unpleasant symptoms.

The potential for bias was great. In selecting patients for studies we looked at patients from a variety of sources. Many were already patients of our clinic but as word spread we received referrals from far and wide, including self-referrals. Maintaining criteria for studies was difficult at times and many patients had to be rejected.

During our studies I learnt of another study (of a different drug for pain) where the research team had offered patients on long waiting lists for a pain clinic appointment the opportunity to participate in the clinical trial in the meantime. What patient would not want to try something as soon as possible for pain relief? This seemed not only to exploit the vulnerability of desperate patients but also to introduce a considerable potential for bias.

One of the questions I have always asked patients participating in our clinical trials is to identify other household members. In particular I have had concerns over teenagers who might be tempted to use such cannabis medication recreationally. However, some clinicians considered this type of questioning to be intrusive and unethical. I have also suggested to patients that they do not tell the whole neighbourhood of their participation in the study to avoid them becoming a target for burglary. The importance of this sort of advice was recently highlighted when the son of one of the patients of our pain clinic recently died after using several tablets of his mother's slow-release morphine 'recreationally' whilst she was out for the night.

In studying cannabis as a medicine we had to decide what our advice should be on driving. Whilst the law gives general advice we had to be specific and realistic. Making patients aware of the risks and their responsibilities has always been our practice. However, the level of advice has been much greater than that given when other, licensed psychoactive drugs are routinely prescribed.

PROBLEMS OCCURRING DURING TRIALS

In starting clinical trials we were fortunate in having a huge body of data to reassure us about the safety of the drug. Not only was there a large body of data from animal research conducted over the preceding 30 years but also extensive anecdotal data. Furthermore, cannabis had been used recreationally over millennia and there was not one substantiated death directly due to the direct effect of the drug. The evidence on the potential for dependency seemed to be low with no significant withdrawal syndrome. Therefore the worries over potential harm were much less than they would have been if this were a totally new chemical being used in humans for the first time.

However, there had been concerns over the potential risk of psychosis emerging and for significant cognitive dysfunction particularly in the heavy user. Over the last 10 years some epidemiological data has been brought together and intensively studied. The significant outcome is that there is an association between occurrence of psychosis in adolescents and recreational smoking of cannabis. Whilst causality has not been shown, opinions get so polarised that rational debate and discussion becomes difficult. Because of the prevalence of often ill-informed articles in the press on the subject, patients have had to be extensively briefed on this. As a result, all studies and off-label use of medicinal cannabis have excluded all patients with a history of drug and alcohol dependency, psychosis and other major psychiatric illness. Unsurprisingly perhaps, such effects have not been seen after such use of medicinal cannabis (with the exception of organic psychosis secondary to physical disease, e.g. severe pyelonephritis, advancing cognitive dysfunction secondary to MS, etc.).

DEATHS: EXPECTED AND UNEXPECTED

About two and a half years after the start of out trials of medicinal cannabis, one of our earliest subjects died unexpectedly. We had seen him a few days before and, knowing him well, had observed no unusual features. In fact quite the reverse; his life had dramatically improved and he now had a partner and a baby daughter. At post-mortem death from a large overdose of amitriptyline was diagnosed. A past history of overdoses when younger also emerged (he had never revealed this to us). However, there were some bizarre features of his death that led to police investigations. Eventually the coroner recorded a verdict of accidental death unrelated to use of medicinal cannabis but the death was reported to the Medicines and Healthcare Products Regulatory Agency (MHRA) as a matter of course. However, I was left with some unhappiness about this outcome as I believe there are still unanswered questions (unrelated to medicinal cannabis use). I have been unable to pursue it further and anyway, I do not feel it would serve any useful interest.

Presenting this episode in public has been difficult. At the time I asked for advice on handling potential media questions on this event from a PR consultant. I recognised that there were potential conflicts of interest between myself as the clinician and the needs of the pharmaceutical company.

A later death befell a person who had become ill during participation in one of the clinical trials at another hospital. The cause of death was multi-factorial and related to coexistent morbidities. Unfortunately the newspaper report in *The Times* on this event mixed the medical use of cannabis with issues of psychosis and recreational cannabis in the young, and the current rumours of a reclassification of cannabis from class C to B. It was clearly nonsense to put three unrelated issues together and reflected the general ill-informed nature of the press coverage. Interpreting what is in the media for the patients in the clinical trials has been a regular necessity.

THE RESULTS OF STUDIES

Our first study on the new cannabis medicine was carried out largely independently and we had no restrictions on what we presented. Based on the information from this, future multi-centre studies were designed and managed by the company. We continued to participate in these and undertook further studies on patients using the medication long term. No restrictions were put on our own independent studies or write-ups, although the company has always been shown our results before publication.

I have also participated in the write-ups of the multi-centre studies. There is a difficulty here in that I had no involvement in the data analysis process. Inevitably this will have consumed huge amounts of man-hours prior to being seen by clinical 'authors' such as myself. Inevitably what I receive is a digest and therefore difficult to dig into to ensure appropriate evaluation.

The studies on MS had proved far more difficult and complex than had been anticipated. Indeed reviews of past studies into the drug management of spasticity showed that there were substantial inadequacies in the outcome measures used which would be unlikely to pass scrutiny today. The current studies have proved difficult in assessing subjective data from heterogeneous groups of patients.

A study I was lead investigator on yielded equivocal results but was rejected for publication. This may reflect the wishes of editors of journals to prefer studies with positive or negative outcomes. However, the results were presented as posters at international meetings.

Undoubtedly many patients achieved a good level of benefit for their pain from the use of the trial drug when many previous treatments had failed. This led me to ask some questions. First, are the same standard methods demanded for evaluating drugs appropriate for every condition from hypertension and diabetes through to pain and spasticity, etc.? The evaluation of pain especially in MS, which is highly heterogeneous and complex in aetiology and symptomatology, is very different from measuring blood sugar levels. The cost and the difficulties in conducting such studies nowadays make this an important ethical question. Furthermore, when patients get substantial relief of pain, is it ethical just to discontinue treatment at the end of the trial?

A further ethical issue arose. I was asked by a high-ranking specialist journal to review a paper on the use of the same drug that my own team was helping to investigate. However, we had not participated in this particular study. I informed the editor of my conflict of interest and he accepted this whilst still requesting my review because of my knowledge of the field. I believe I was harsher in my comments and criticisms than the other reviewer as I was able to pick out gaps in the presentation. However, I also needed to ensure that my impartiality was seen to be as good as I could make it!

USING AN UNLICENSED DRUG

When we were studying the cannabis extract it was anticipated that a licence would be issued by about 2004. However, this did not occur but many patients with intractable symptoms wanted to try the drug. Our knowledge of the drug and experience in its use enabled us to give patients the opportunity. The MHRA had concluded that the drug was of the required standard in terms of formulation and that it was safe. The stumbling block for the regulators was the level of statistical evidence that they required.

A problem of funding immediately arose. Some patients could afford to pay and accepted this. Other patients we treated on a compassionate basis using funds bequeathed to our clinic for patient care. However, deciding who should have medication paid for has been a difficult decision.

In time, if the drug achieves a licence, then the local therapeutics advisory group will want advice on the appropriateness of the drug for clinical use. On the one hand, I will have the experience, but, on the other hand, I may be a very biased enthusiast. My long history of working with the manufacturers could count against my opinion. Yet I want the best treatment for my patients. Furthermore I have to consider what my action should be if the regulators or the National Institute for Health and Clinical Excellence (NICE) decide against its routine use. Do I mount a campaign in the media for its use, a method which has already been widely used for other drugs?

THE MEDIA

The development of cannabis as a medicine has been a 'sexy' subject for the media since the mid-1990s. Radio, newspapers, magazines, TV, etc. have all shown repeated interest. Many journalists have been referred to me for an opinion when news of research results or adverse effects has emerged and I also seemed to become an unofficial reference point for the British Medical Association.

In the early days I found myself being approached for an opinion on the medical use as an add-on to the debate about recreational cannabis (and other drug use) that has been a continual political issue. These were usually live, studio discussions, often degenerating into haranguing. On one occasion I found myself on the daytime *Kilroy* show (over a different issue) and vowed never to do this type of programme again. However, I soon decided to refuse to discuss the medical issue in the context of the recreational debate. The medical use of diamorphine is never discussed at the same time and place as the illicit use. However, even now, I occasionally get caught out. I gave an interview on our research programme recently to one of our local TV stations. Back in the newsroom this was merged with a breaking regional story about the discovery of a large cannabis 'factory' being run by Vietnamese immigrants.

Fortunately, amongst the sound bites there has been a steady stream of journalists (radio, TV, magazines, newspapers) wanting to do a 'serious' story on the subject. Trying to define the media's approach has often been a difficult problem. Watching what I say has been hard work. I have winced on occasions as I have seen my words from an unguarded moment set in print by journalists wanting a more visceral comment on the situation ('lives that are crap' or 'a load of bollocks') or just the description, 'a rumpled, 59-year-old anaesthesiologist'!

I have often been asked by journalists to provide them with patients to interview for radio, TV and print media. Inevitably I have selected patients who have had good benefit from treatment and are willing to talk. The journalist therefore does not get a cross-section and merely focuses on the success stories. Caring for the patient has always been a priority though, along with maintaining confidentiality. Therefore setting the ground rules for any interactions has been essential.

Some of the media interest has been arranged in connection with the PR organisation used by GW Pharmaceuticals. I have been offered up to journalists as an 'independent' clinician, experienced in the field. In dealing with the PR manager, I wonder sometimes whether the relationship has been symbiotic, parasitic, infective or even mutagenic.

MISINFORMATION IN THE MEDIA

As the media became more interested in the research into cannabis extract pieces of incorrect information started to circulate. For example, it was repeatedly reported that the materials under study had had all the psychoactive elements removed and therefore would have no significant adverse effects on the brain. The perception was that this was somehow 'sanitised' cannabis which could not cause a 'high'. This was not true. The research we were undertaking was on the active ingredients of the cannabis plant that, if given in sufficient quantity, would be as effective as any illicitly obtained cannabis plant material.

Obviously it was of benefit to the pharmaceutical company to allow this myth to continue as it put the product in a good light with regulators, politicians and others. However, when faced with a direct question on this issue from a journalist I found myself needing to correct this misinformation. Over the years I have realised the importance of dispelling the ignorance about cannabis particularly as people have very polarised views on the subject, often based on little real evidence or understanding.

POLITICIANS: WHOSE AGENDA?

In the 1994 a group of professionals, members of the public and politicians met with three ministers at the Ministry of Health to try to find ways to take forward the study of cannabis as a medicine. Whilst there was sympathy shown, the regulators seemed impervious to suggestions of change.

By 1997 there was a growing public and professional call to allow such studies to be initiated and a further meeting took place in December. Again there seemed no simple way through, nor any desire to change. However, one of the participants who attended realised that the way forward was to work within the regulations. The outcome five months later was the establishment of GW Pharmaceuticals to investigate extracts of plant cannabis. This fulfilled the politicians' wish to see the medicinal and recreational issues separated. Furthermore they felt comfortable that the target group of patients would be those with MS. In the US patients with HIV/AIDS were the active group promoting cannabis use as a medicine. This was probably much less acceptable to the establishment and was seen to be the thin end of the wedge to allow personal cultivation. Hence the US is at least eight years behind the UK in terms of clinical research.

Unfortunately the research has proved very difficult. MS is one of the hardest diseases to study symptom control in. Whilst the new cannabis medicine proved safe and of high quality, the necessary statistical standard was not quite achieved. A pragmatic and humanitarian response from regulators would have allowed use of the medicine. At the time of writing, the new drug has 11 years of clinical study (and millennia of human use) but has only just received its licence. During this time reports on the possible adverse psychiatric effects from recreational use emerged.

The ongoing political difficulties with the classification of cannabis have muddied the waters especially as the opinions of independent experts on the long-term strategies for recreational use have been ignored. It is a simple step to consider that there has possibly been a lack of enthusiasm by politicians to get the medicine established. The MPs have gone very quiet whilst patients continue to suffer.

A more recent meeting between two ministers and myself and an MP made no headway. Moreover I came out confused and not knowing really whose agenda I had been supporting: The MPs? The pharmaceutical company? My own? My patients?

FINANCIAL INTERESTS

GW Pharmaceuticals floated on the stock exchange as a public company. Some have estimated that the potential market for cannabinoids is over $1 billion and the opportunity to buy in to the fortunes of the company has always been there. However, I opted not to invest recognising that to do so would have a negative impact on my independence.

I have often been approached by friends and colleagues for advice on investment in GW Pharma. I believe that I have kept such advice to what is in the public domain and to what can be generalised across the field. My main concern has been to avoid revealing any insider information on the results of unpublished trial data.

However, there were three other sources of financing that involved me. First, my research team has received ongoing support funding for any commercial research undertaken and this is of major importance to the survival of the team. However, I refused to be paid personally ensuring that all related work was done over and above my NHS contract. Secondly, I have received occasional consultancy fees from GW Pharma just as I have from other pharmaceutical companies over the years. Thirdly, I have been funded to speak at various meetings, academic and teaching. The payments have been for expenses and preparation of presentations. A presentation might take 12 hours to prepare. Such payments did not make up for the small private practice which I discontinued.

I have declared all such income to my employer. As a result, when I was interviewed by a *Guardian* newspaper journalist recently who had obtained a copy of my hospital's 'register of interests' and wanted to ask about money I had received from another pharmaceutical company, I was able to account for the work I had done and explain the fee I had received. The article on fees and hospitality received by doctors made the front page but without comment on my own activities. The use of the Freedom of Information Act may reveal the extent of any doctor's involvement with industry. The need to be able to demonstrate that fees are justifiable and ethical may become increasing frequent.

It is becoming a requirement for statements of financial disclosure to be made for speakers at conferences and for authors of papers submitted to journals. Such statements are important for the audience in their evaluation of the information presented. In teaching or lecturing I have always prepared my own presentations and insisted on editorial independence in deciding and commenting on whatever material I have used. I have never had this refused.

MY NHS EMPLOYER

My NHS employer has always been aware of all my activities, both research and extramural. The hospital requires compliance with its register of interests. I use annual leave where I believe that any extra-mural activity cannot be justified as part of my NHS work.

In keeping my employers briefed I have recognised that the hospital has benefited from the publicity that such clinical trials have brought and has given active support – some explicit and some that my intuition tells me have been behind the scenes. Furthermore, the NHS has benefited from the treatment of patients, and patients themselves have benefited from increased and effective treatment of their conditions.

CONCLUSIONS

The reality nowadays is that only the pharmaceutical industry has the ability to develop, produce and market new drugs. The industry needs knowledgeable clinicians to advise them, to undertake research, to educate other doctors and to help promote its products. Recently I have been teaching groups of Canadian doctors about the practical aspects of treating patients with cannabis-based medicines as I have over 10 years of clinical experience.

I have attempted to maintain my independence although it has been difficult at times to identify the ethical boundaries. It is reasonable to believe that I have been of use to the companies I have been involved with. So, have I been manipulated or used; have I maintained my integrity; has the bundling been effective or have I crossed the line? That is for you, the reader, to decide.

CHAPTER 5

What are pain clinics for?

Ian Yellowlees

INTRODUCTION

Generally, care for those in pain is provided by the local family doctor, and only a small minority reach a specialist pain service. Those that do arrive at the door of a specialist service do so with a wide variety of pain problems and other medical issues, but also, and perhaps most importantly, with expectations and (usually) misunderstandings. This is not surprising. Pain destroys people's lives, relationships, and sense of self and over the years sufferers develop hopes, fears and beliefs about their problems that often cause as much difficulty as the reported pain.

It seems obvious that a specialist pain service should treat the patient's pain. Unfortunately, because of the complexity of pain and the interactions of psychosocial factors and physical factors this is not often possible, at least in the direct way that patients may hope for. Most patients attending a specialist service have had pain problems for many years, have seen many different specialists and have tried many different treatments before they arrive at the clinic. By definition, all these interventions have failed to treat the pain problem. So what is there left for a specialist clinic to do? What *do* patients expect from such a service?

EXPECTATIONS

The answer looks different depending on whether you are staff or patient. At a superficial level patients would of course like attendance at a pain clinic to result in a cure for their pain at an acceptable cost in terms of side effects. Some hope for this magic cure even though they know, deep down, that such magic is not available. Others come to a clinic still convinced that there must be a cure, if only they can find the right doctor. All patients have also heard, or misheard, numerous explanations of the problem, and have had to endure the psychological effect of numerous failed treatments. Staff, on the other hand, generally have lower, or perhaps just different, expectations. They usually hope to increase a patient's functional capacity, and, perhaps, to reduce the pain *a bit*. So the initial consultation often starts with an imbalance of expectation.

Thus the first role of a pain service must be to engage the patient and manage expectations.

Most specialist clinics explicitly recognise this as part of their role, and try to help patients move from unrealistic expectations and hopes of a cure, towards a more holistic view of the problems. Most clinics would accept that if this can be achieved then attention can be focused on moving forward with the problem rather than looking back to what might have been.

Unfortunately reaching this goal may also result in a temporary undermining of the patient's beliefs, opinions and hopes, and thus must be undertaken slowly and with care. It is a two-way process and to follow this route patients must be willing to look at and re-evaluate all of these aspects. But what if a patient does not want, or feels unable to face, the truth of the situation (as portrayed by the specialist)?

If patients have no expectations that the service can achieve anything, or are reluctant to follow the path the specialist thinks is the best, how much should the possible benefit of working with the service be talked up in order to engage them? This is dodgy ground from an ethical perspective. Talking up the possible benefit requires us to be reasonably sure that there are benefits to be had. How good is the advice we give? A cool critical look at what clinics actually achieve tends to be rather uncomfortable for those whose jobs depend on the existence of pain clinics. Evidence-based guidelines are singularly lacking in the pain world, and much of our treatment is based on anecdote, experience and population-level studies. Many of the studies that have been done have looked at depressingly short follow-up periods, often less than one year, which seems to be rather a brief period of time given that many of these patients have had pain for a decade or more. Of course we must remain aware that maybe the patients are right, perhaps a cure *will* be developed, or perhaps the referral *is* a waste of time. Such an open-minded approach is not comfortable for professionals. Maybe all that pain services can really do is promise to try to help, using all that we know about pain, with the (slightly) comforting thought that most of us working in these specialist services probably know more about pain than most family doctors.

Trying to help a patient with chronic pain is therefore a partnership, and it may be useful here to explore the realm of the doctor/patient relationship and the concept of the 'patient's work'.

The patient's work

The concept that the patient has responsibilities, i.e. has work to do and a role to perform has been explored by others. In *The Healer's Power* Howard Brody[1] noted that a doctor and patient must collaborate in some way for treatment to be successful. But if collaboration is required for a treatment to have the best chance of success, clearly an assessment of the patient and the work they are expecting and willing to do should determine our treatment plans. However, professionals would then have to accept that the treatment plan arrived at may not be what they as specialists regard as best management. The agreed treatment plan may not even follow established guidelines. This will require pain service staff to be flexible and willing to compromise their own initial ideas of what is 'best' for the patient in favour of what is the best that can be achieved given the patients 'work ethos'. They will need to accept that this is, in this particular situation, the best outcome.

At first glance this concept may seem strange, but it is perhaps little different from a physician knowing the 'right' antibiotic for a particular infection, but also being able to accept that the patient may not want any antibiotic at all – a decision that could have serious health consequences – and that this may be the 'best' outcome.

Three roles or models (and associated work) are often used to describe different patient/doctor relationships, and much has been written about this and many research projects have been based around these concepts.

For our purposes in the pain clinic it may be helpful to consider the three models.

➤ *The dependant patient*
  This classic model of care is instinctively embraced by physicians and patients alike. The patient has a role, and this role involves the patient in obligations just as any other role in society. By convention the sick person is exempt from normal social roles, and is deemed to be in some way not responsible for their condition.

  Equally, there is an obligation upon the person that they should try to get well and that they should seek help from competent medical professionals.

  For some patients this appeals strongly, probably because it relates to previous experiences of the caring parent.

  Doctors also like it because it calls for unquestioning acceptance from the patient. However, this kind of model seems to be based on the assumption that the illness is likely to be treatable or at least of short duration.

➤ *The 'take charge' patient*
  In this model, patients take part in the process of thinking about choices and making decisions. If they do not, the treatment process cannot start. The work required of the patient is to become informed *and then choose*. This is the role championed by some healthcare organisations seeking to create a patient driven service.

This role has the potential advantage that it may help to restore a degree of control and self-esteem in a patient. The 'learned helplessness' model of depression much talked about in the pain world describes how patients come over time to see their situation as hopeless because of the repeated failure of treatments. The model emphasises the importance of active control over one's environment as a key to maintaining self-esteem in the face of adversity or failure.

➤ *The conversationalist patient*
In this model, the relationship can be likened to a conversation, the eventual aim of which is for the patient to develop self-understanding and use his illness and suffering to create something useful for the future management of the problem. The work required of the patient is a willingness to engage in a constructive conversation that leads somewhere, and use the result to help manage life problems.

A little thought reveals that trying to shift a patient to accept a role different from the one they naturally take up may require considerable input and time. *Imposing* a particular role is likely to lead to failure and an unsatisfactory encounter for both staff and patient. Unfortunately with the pressure of waiting lists, clinic time and targets it is all too easy to impose on the patient and *tell* them what they 'must' do to benefit from the service input – 'take this drug', or 'go to that exercise class'. Classical medical education of the early to mid-20th century often assumed a dependent patient, and many services round the world have been developed by physicians with such a classical upbringing. Small wonder then that what research is available often suggests that pain clinic results are patchy at best.

However, accepting the concept of these roles also brings problems. In a long-term condition such as chronic pain, the *dependant patient* consumes resources, often for many years. Without a cure the best that can be achieved is likely to be oft-repeated temporary relief. The resource input is open ended.

The *take control patient* has to understand complex medical issues and decide on treatment in a situation where they may be almost overwhelmed by the pain problem. Perhaps these are the patients who need 'window of opportunity' injections and drugs to give them temporary relief in which to learn, understand and choose. Once a decision is made, the outcome is, at least in part, their choice.

The *conversationalist* also consumes resources, as the process of self-development and construction of psychological management tools is often long and complex. However, unlike the situation with the *dependant* patient, it is not open ended; the aim is self-management.

If we regard all three roles as in some way ethically equal, and acceptance of them and cooperation with them as important for successful outcome, they need to be recognised at the start of management. In all three role models the patient has work to do, and management or treatment of the pain problem by a specialist service needs to include supervision and monitoring of the patient's work. If the work is not done (by the patient or the professionals) the treatment plan will fail.

In some healthcare situations there is a fourth patient role. *The uncooperative patient.* Sometimes the patient only comes along at another's request (the family doctor, insurance company, family or friends) and thinks the referral is a waste of time. In effect these patients do not want to be there at all. This is a difficult one for specialist services. Should we respect their wishes and just say goodbye, or respect the implied wish of the (formal or informal) referrer that we try to engage the patient in working with the pain service? Has the patient, by turning up on the day, implicitly asked for treatment?

So where have we got to? At the start, managing expectations, beliefs and hopes appeared to be a simple first step in the service offered by a specialist pain clinic, but this actually turns out to be a complex, two-way process. The expectations of the patient have to be integrated with those of the physician, and need to take account of the nature of the work the patient is prepared to undertake.

But let us move on and suppose that all is going well. The patient and clinician have (implicitly) agreed common expectations for what the service is trying to do, and have managed to establish a concept (even if this is just a mutual understanding) of the roles to be taken by each party. The next job for the specialist service would seem to be to treat the patient.

WHAT TREATMENTS SHOULD BE OFFERED?

All medical services have limited resources, and a seemingly endless stream of patients requiring help. Should the specialist pain clinic try to provide whatever is best for treating a patient? Recall that the argument developed so far is based around the concept that a collaboration between doctor and patient is required in order to achieve the best result for the patient, and that this will require an investigation and understanding of the patient's work ethos. The argument implies that there is a perfectly reasonable ethical justification for managing a long term condition in a *dependant type* doctor/patient relationship with repeated short-term treatments (e.g. some types of injections or drugs). But it also implies an equal justification for long-term psychological treatment for a *conversationalist* patient seeking meaning and understanding – particularly as the aim of this treatment is to develop tools that the patient can eventually use to self-manage the problem.

Or perhaps a specialist service should try to do the most good for the most people. In the major trauma situation it seems to be accepted that available resources are used to help those who have a good chance of survival for modest resource input, rather than treating those who have a small chance of survival even with major input. This is known as triage. If this is acceptable in trauma, should the same ideas apply to a pain service? Although this seems logical at a non-emotional level, pain services have significant problems with this philosophy, partly because we are notoriously bad at assessing prognosis. In trauma victims, the major problems tend to be more obvious in the early stages, and triage decisions are perhaps easier. Even if we wanted to target resources within a pain service towards those most likely to benefit, we do not usually have the ability to select the targets reliably. So most clinics in the end try to help all comers even though it is clearly not going to be realistic to fulfil both of these objectives – to accept 'all comers', *and* to give them whatever is necessary for treatment (even if we actually knew with any certainty what that was).

So perhaps the next question to be considered when wondering what pain clinics are for is to look at who gets what and why. Is the division of the pot in any way logical or fair?

DIVISION OF THE RESOURCE POT

Pain services generally come under the umbrella of acute services because of the historical link with anaesthetics. This is often unhelpful because the management of pain is a *process*, not an *event* like giving an anaesthetic or repairing a hernia.

I suspect that few pain clinicians have, prior to fighting for resources, consciously developed a coherent ethical structure on which to base their work taking due account of the patient's work ethos and the long-term financial consequences of providing various types of treatment. For example, most clinics shy away from providing long-term psychodynamic therapy over a period of years (perhaps best management for a *conversationalist* patient) but are happy to provide intermittent injections over a period of years (to the *dependant* patient).

If we accept the ideas presented above we must conclude that such practice is discriminatory and unethical. It also makes no financial sense. At 2009 prices in the healthcare service where I work, an X-ray guided injection costs about £500 and a one-hour psychology session about £100. So if a *dependant* type patient receives two injections per year the cost is £1000 per year, potentially for many years. A *conversationalist* type patient might need a session of psychology every two weeks for two years before permanent discharge to self-management. This would be a total cost of £5000, equivalent to just the first five years of support for the *dependant* patient.

The ethical and financial arguments in favour of a broad-based treatment provision seem good. But now we come to the types of physician, and their expectations for their role in society and in life.

It is a saying in the pain world that clinicians come in two (prejudiced) types, 'needle-jockeys' (those that favour treatment by injections and other invasive techniques) and 'tea and sympathy brigade' (those that take an holistic, more psychological approach). Too often who gets what in a specialist pain clinic is governed in large part by staff prejudices or preferences –often justified as 'experience'. This is not a simple problem to fix. Just trying to get a balance of the two extremes of staff type is not enough to ensure ethical, clinical and financial probity in a clinic if the clinic has not developed a coherent philosophy as discussed above. Even if it has, the staff need to recognise the patient types and accept that they as an individual may not be the right staff member to manage an individual patient. This is a difficult managerial problem and requires a great deal of honesty from the staff.

There is obviously a place for clinics that specialise in certain treatments, or only provide a few treatments, but to be morally justifiable this must be explicit and does not obviate these clinics from the need to understand what it is that they are doing.

CONCLUSIONS

So what is a pain clinic for? In trying to answer this question I have highlighted some of the ethical problems that are faced (or should be faced) by specialist pain services when designing the service and working with individual patients. But in doing so I have perhaps skirted around the actual question of what they are *for*. This is perhaps because there is no simple answer, and all that can be said is that the specialist pain clinic exists primarily to help patients with their pain problem in the broadest sense. Pain is a very complex phenomenon, and chronic pain involves all aspects of a person's life. Whilst in the occasional patient it may be possible to achieve great benefit by prescribing a simple pain killer, helping patients with their pain problem usually involves the development of cooperation and understanding between the staff and the patient in order to achieve a plan for the future. If this process is successful, and the plan achieved, this will be the 'best' outcome, although it will not necessarily be what guidelines or a staff members' prejudices might consider the best. Achieving this 'best' outcome requires staff (and patients) to face up to, own up to and work with their own characteristics as a person, and their wants and prejudices. Sadly, we all too often see professionals pursuing their own interests and treatment prejudices, often to the detriment of the patient.

Perhaps there is hope for the future. Modern medical education is very aware of the issues noted in this chapter and many of the new doctors coming through try hard to work out what is genuinely best for the patient and then help them to achieve it whether or not this fits with their own particular interest.

REFERENCE

1   Brody H. *The Healer's Power.* New Haven, CT: Yale University Press; 1993.

CHAPTER 6

Management of the complex patient in the pain clinic

Diana Brighouse

How do we deal with the complex/difficult/end-of-the road patient in the pain clinic?

What do we mean by 'difficult'? Doctors make casual reference to the difficult patient, the heart sink patient and even more pejoratively the demanding and manipulative patient.

This chapter will explore not only how we might manage this group of patients but also why medicine tends to categorise them in this way.

DUALISM

Throughout the last century Western medicine has adhered to a broadly dualistic Cartesian philosophy of mind/body split. This has been accompanied by an increasing trend towards reductionism – stated simplistically this is a belief that the explanation for everything can eventually be discovered (and by inference treated). Reductionism is of course much more complex than this, and philosophers identify at least three core types of reductionism in biology; ontological, methodological and epistemic.[1] For the purposes of this chapter reductionism is taken to mean ontological reductionism, the idea that an organism is composed of molecules and their interactions, and can be entirely explained in those terms.

Evidence-based medicine is predicated on a reductionist system in which everything can be reduced to measurable units that can then be compared. This works well in a systems-based economy, which is the underlying philosophy of British National Health Service (NHS) management. Patients become units in the system; each patient consists of a number of component units and the job of the clinicians is to diagnose and treat the dysfunctional component. Treatments are compared using quantitative data and the most cost-effective treatment is approved. The over arching goal is efficiency; targets are set to improve efficiency (and thus save money) year on year. The NHS has adopted the 'Lean' model, developed by the car manufacturer Toyota, with the intention of 'improving flow and eliminating waste'.

> Lean brings into many industries, including healthcare, new concepts, tools and methods that have been effectively utilised to improve process flow. Tools that address workplace organisation, standardisation, visual control and elimination of non-value added steps are applied to improve flow, eliminate waste and exceed customer expectations.[2]

Within such a system the clinician also becomes a component with a defined task, working within a circumscribed framework described by protocols and guidelines. Individualism is discouraged and there is a background awareness of the threat of referral to management or professional regulating bodies. The emphasis is on productivity, efficiency and working 'smarter'.

Such reductionism encourages focus on the body as a machine, concentrating on diagnosis and repair of faulty or malfunctioning parts. The mind is seen as another component of the machine that has historically been managed with a wide-ranging spectrum of treatments, but over recent years there has been considerable interest in targeted drug therapy that conforms to the systems model.

Attempts to integrate mind and body have been made, particularly in the areas of chronic pain and liaison psychiatry, with the adoption of the biopsychosocial rather than the biomedical model. This model recognises that the patient's psyche and their social circumstances are significant contributors to their presenting biological symptoms, the implication being that management of the patient's complaint will involve psychological and social management. However, for the chronic pain patient (and many patients in primary care) psychological treatment now equates to cognitive behavioural therapy (CBT), either on an individual basis or in groups through pain management programmes. There is also a danger that the clinician falls back into the trap of dualism and approaches the patient with the concept that the pain is all psychological.

CBT claims evidence-based efficacy and has become a panacea for a multitude of conditions. It undoubtedly has its place in both primary and secondary care, but it is far from a universal magic bullet. CBT conforms well to a reductionist approach; it is to a large extent protocol driven and its evidence base is a product of quantitative data. Quantitative data are highly relevant to a systems-based model but arguably not widely applicable in a more holistic model of care. How is a numerical value given to a patient's suffering, to their relationship with their partner or children?

THE EXPLANATORY GAP

The reductive model has served western medicine well, and our scientifically orientated society acknowledges the pre-eminence of reductionism. However, the question of how to measure suffering illustrates a limitation of the model that has been widely discussed by philosophers. There is a range of experiences related to abstract human consciousness that cannot apparently be explained by physical processes.

The explanatory gap proposes that there is:

> ... a gap of coherent meaningful information describing and accounting for qualities and characteristics of consciousness content, processes, and states that is explainable to a logical level of understanding.[3]

The concept was first proposed by Joseph Levine in 1983 and has been debated extensively since then.[4] The failure to explain consciousness in terms of physical substrates is seen by some as a practical problem of the current limitations of human understanding – i.e. the gap is closable, whereas others believe that in principle the gap can never be closed. There is an enormous literature pertaining to consciousness studies and the explanatory gap.

The French existential philosopher and psychotherapist Julia Kristeva coined the term intertextuality in response to her study of semiotics. She suggests that the meaning of a text is not a simple two-way process between the author and the reader, but that meaning derives from a multiplicity of other texts. Intertextuality has subsequently been used in much wider contexts, and the intertextual space could be considered analogous to the transpersonal space referred to by some psychotherapists. Transpersonal psychology takes into account not only that which is obvious in the here and now, but also that which lies within the realms of the spiritual or higher consciousness. 'The transpersonal relationship is the timeless facet of the psychotherapeutic relationship, which is impossible to describe, but refers to the spiritual dimension of the healing relationship.'[5] Both 'intertextual' and 'transpersonal' are attempts to define the indefinable, that which falls into the remit of the explanatory gap.

Although the relationship between therapist and patient is recognised in behavioural therapies it is not considered to be the focus of treatment (any more than in the majority of patient/doctor consultations in secondary care – and increasingly in primary care). However, work in the intertextual or transpersonal space is work that occurs primarily in the non verbal communication between doctor and patient. Psychotherapists working non-behaviourally use themselves as the primary therapeutic tool – it is the relationship between the therapist and the patient that is paramount.

Many pain patients arrive in the clinic having been subjected to sequential encounters with reductive medicine. They have frequently been referred into secondary care by their GPs with a request for assistance in diagnosing a cause for the pain. It is unlikely that the new patient in the chronic pain clinic will have had an extended consultation with their GP or another consultant, although they have often been regular attendees in primary care and may have accumulated several hours of consultation time over a lengthy period. The greater the number of brief consultations with different healthcare providers the greater is the opportunity for the patient to become confused, receive mixed or even conflicting messages about their symptoms, and the more likely the patient is to pursue the elusive diagnosis of the 'cause' for their pain, with the implication of definitive cure.

The corollary of this scenario is that the healthcare provider, educated in a reductive model and urged towards 'lean' practice, will also be seeking the dysfunctional component to rectify, and when he or she fails to find it one of two possibilities may occur. Either the practitioner feels that he or she has failed and introjects this sense of failure, or that he or she projects the sense of failure into the patient. The patient may then non-verbally receive the message that he or she is hopeless, or that somehow he or she is to blame for the pain. Another manifestation of this sense of failure is the complaint that 'my doctor said it was all in my mind'. This is a direct result of body/mind dualism – the unwritten statement that if no physical cause can be found for the patient's symptoms then the symptoms must be a product of the imagination. It is an unfortunate fact that even in the 21st century there are doctors who believe that pain from, for example, a broken leg, is more 'real' than chronic pain without a diagnosable physical cause, and that the latter pain does not merit treatment with strong analgesics (even if they are effective). Postulating that a patient with chronic pain may be presenting physical expression of emotional trauma does not deny the reality of the physical pain, nor the neurobiological changes that accompany the pain.

Many chronic pain patients can be more effectively managed with early intervention and good multidisciplinary care, but conventional pain clinic biopsychosocial models of care can still be quite reductive in their approach. The emphasis is on multidisciplinary care which again means that the patient may see several different healthcare professionals, and even when there is a unified strategy and message some patients will readily take away any minor differences, and grasp at any opportunity of pursuing a physical 'cause' for their pain. Patients entering the pain management programme receive group CBT, which may not meet their needs. Some patients are deemed unsuitable for the pain management programme and may well then be seen to have reached the end of the line, whilst those that have been through the programme and have either not improved or failed to maintain improvement may well be considered to have failed all available treatment. What then can be done to help this group of patients?

Many of these 'end of road' patients fall into a grey area between mental health and physical medicine, with neither group of specialists enthusiastic about taking over their care. I would argue that it is increasingly the role of the pain clinic to care for this group, especially as much of the historic work of pain clinics has either become less frequent as a result of NICE guidelines (non-specialist interventional work) or can be devolved into primary care teams overseen by consultants. I believe that the pain consultant should be a specialist of intertextual/transpersonal medicine, working non-reductively. It is important to emphasise that this does not preclude the use of drugs as part of the package of care; these patients have 'real' pain and the symptoms need to be treated appropriately from the pharmaceutical armamentarium available. However, the primary therapeutic tool will be the healthcare provider.

CASE STUDIES

The following case studies (fictional patients with details from a variety of clinic patients) illustrate this way of working.

Susan

Susan is 48 years old and married with two children. She has chronic abdominal pain and was referred by her GP to the gastroenterologists. She has been extensively investigated and has also been seen by the gynaecologists and a colorectal surgeon. No identifiable cause has been found for her pain. She is unable to work, has extreme difficulty in looking after her children and is increasingly dependent on her husband to help with running the house. She uses a wheelchair on occasions. She takes large doses of morphine which only partially relieve her pain.

Susan was referred to the pain clinic by the gastroenterologists who said that they were unable to find any reason for her pain.

At initial consultation Susan was defensive and unforthcoming. She understood that she had come to the clinic to be weaned off her morphine, and told me that she had been told that her pain was in her mind.

During this first one-hour consultation little further history was obtained beyond that already in her medical records. A further appointment was made and no adjustment was made to her medication.

Over a period of three further 50-minute appointments Susan divulged that she had been sexually abused by her father as a child, and that she had also been forced to witness her father beating her mother on

(continued)

a regular basis. She had once tried to tell a teacher about this but had been told not to make up such wicked stories. She had been raped as a young woman and escaped the family home as soon as she could. She had never talked about any of her early life experiences as she felt that she would not be believed. She felt a mixture of shame and guilt, and had never been able to tell her husband what had happened to her.

Susan entered weekly psychodynamic psychotherapy and over the course of a year was able to explore the impact of her childhood experiences, and through the therapeutic relationship was able to gain some sense of self-worth. At the end of the year she felt strong enough to join a therapeutic group for survivors of sexual abuse. She had reduced her analgesic consumption significantly and was able to contribute a little more to running the house.

Pamela

Pamela is a lady in her 40s who presented to the pain clinic with chest pain. She had also been extensively investigated by other consultants in secondary care, having been referred sequentially by a number of different GPs in the large practice with which she was registered. She had a complex social history which was documented (with conflicting detail) in her medical records. Her pain had been present since she was assaulted whilst serving a prison sentence. It was very clear from the numerous letters in her medical records that she had exhausted the patience and interest of each doctor who had seen her.

Pamela was taking high doses of antidepressants and using fentanyl patches to (unsuccessfully) manage her pain. She was hostile and verbally aggressive at the initial consultation, saying that she was wasting her time, and that she wasn't a 'nutter' and that her pain was not in her head. The first consultation consisted of listening to her complaints about her previous treatment and about her GPs, and trying to gain her confidence.

Pamela had monthly appointments for nine months before stating that she felt able to trust her pain consultant, at which point she started to talk about her family history. After a further six months she entered weekly psychotherapy for a year. She had a history of childhood sexual abuse from her father and two uncles, and also from her mother. She had run away from home and from school and had twice been placed in care; on one of these occasions she had been abused by a care worker after telling him about her home experiences. During her time in prison

(continued)

she had been propositioned by a prison officer. It is not surprising that after these experiences she felt unable to trust anyone, especially figures of authority.

The main aim of psychotherapy for Pamela was to enable her to develop a meaningful and eventually trusting relationship with another human being – something that she had never experienced. This was not going to be easy and one year of therapy could only lay down the foundations of relationship, but hopefully enabled Pamela to start to value herself.

Barbara

Barbara is a petite 59-year-old referred with chronic abdominal pain. She had been investigated for pain and persistent low weight by the gastroenterologists and was also under the care of the community mental health team for anxiety and depression. She was convinced that she had a physical cause for her pain and was very worried that an underlying cancer remained undiagnosed. She expressed unhappiness at her referral as she was aware that the pain clinic would not be offering her further investigations. However, she was receptive to the idea that her pain could in part be related to her anxiety, and agreed to a series of consultations to consider this.

Over the course of six 50-minute appointments it emerged that Barbara had had an emotionally abusive first marriage to a perfectionist husband. He had expected her to keep the house in an immaculate condition at the same time as bringing up two small children. She had grown up in a similar household and believed that this was her duty as a wife. Her husband had taunted her about her appearance if she failed 'to come up to scratch' and had refused to touch her during her pregnancies because he found her 'fat and repulsive'. She had gone on crash diets and punishing exercise regimes after the birth of each child. She had maintained a low weight by following a restrictive diet long term, and felt that maintaining her size eight figure was essential for being loved. The marriage ended with the premature death of her husband from a myocardial infarct – a death that Barbara admitted to feeling somehow responsible for. Five years later she remarried and although she says that her new husband is much more relaxed than the first one she accepts that 'keeping up standards' is essential for her.

(continued)

More detailed questioning revealed that Barbara ate a very restricted diet amounting to about 800 kcal daily, and that she had abused laxatives for many years. She had never revealed this to anyone. She was disbelieving but relieved to be told that she had an eating disorder – her belief was that such a diagnosis only occurred in teenagers. She readily agreed to referral to the eating disorder service where she had individual psychotherapy and regular consultations with the dietician.

At pain clinic follow-up one year later Barbara was managing her pain without analgesics, had had no further hospital admissions with pain, and her body mass index had risen from 16.5 to 19.

Frank

Frank is a 64-year-old professional man referred to the pain clinic by his GP. He had severe back pain and had taken early retirement because of this. By the time he was seen in the clinic he was walking with two sticks and using opioid analgesia. He had been investigated by the orthopaedic surgeons and had also attended the back care functional restoration programme. He had received extensive physiotherapy and was conscientious about performing his exercises at home. He tried to get out for a short walk each day and occupied himself with household tasks as his wife was still working. He was articulate and readily admitted that he felt a failure. From his perspective he had failed at work because of taking early retirement, he had failed as a husband because the family income had dropped and his pain had virtually eliminated his libido and he had failed all his doctors because he had not got better.

Frank was unusual it that he asked to enter psychotherapy, and it was agreed that he should have a six-month course. He talked about his experiences at boarding school where he had been bullied consistently, and his inability to form any relationship with his father who was a cold and distant man who had bullied Frank's mother. It became clear that Frank's wife was a domineering and emotionally distant woman who taunted Frank about his failure to be a 'real man' and belittled his work in the house. Frank had been in love with a girl who had been deemed unsuitable by his father, and his subsequent marriage had virtually been arranged by both sets of parents.

Frank responded well to therapy and although his pain did not alter a great deal he became much more able to manage it. He was able to stop his analgesics and by the end of therapy was using only occasional

(continued)

paracetamol. He had hoped to persuade his wife to enter marriage guidance counselling but was unable to do so, and was contemplating marital separation.

Sally

Sally is a 44-year-old woman with shoulder and arm pain that had been present for many years but had become much worse over the preceding three years. She had been investigated by the rheumatologists and orthopaedic surgeons and had been told that she had nothing wrong with her. She had given up work because of the pain and the family was struggling financially, with her husband working overtime to compensate for her loss of earnings. Sally had had eight sessions of CBT and had also been through the pain management programme, and she was upset and frustrated that her pain was still just as bad and that she could not manage it.

Over the course of six months of fortnightly consultations Sally developed a good therapeutic relationship with her pain consultant and was able to talk about the sexual abuse that she had suffered at the hands of her stepfather, which had continued during her engagement to her husband. She had never been able to tell her husband because her stepfather had convinced her that she was 'soiled goods' that nobody would want if they knew that she was 'such a slut'. The apparent trigger for Sally's pain becoming intolerable had been her mother's death.

Sally was eventually able to recognise that her physical pain was linked to her emotional pain and that she needed to address both in order to be able to manage them. She had the opportunity to enter a therapeutic group but felt that she was not ready for this. She really wanted to have weekly psychotherapy but was unable to afford this privately, and there was no NHS availability. The situation was partially resolved by referral to low-cost therapy, although this entailed a lengthy waiting list.

These cases are typical of many patients referred to chronic pain clinics, and will also be familiar to primary care physicians. Sexual and emotional abuse in childhood is extremely common, and the incidence is even higher in patients with mental health problems. It has been reported that 48–61% of chronic pain patients have a history of long-term abuse.[6,7] All types of childhood abuse cause wounds that will eventually manifest themselves physically or mentally. Children grow up learning to establish healthy relationships with themselves and others through attachment to a secure, loving protector – usually the mother and/or father. If the protector is the perpetrator of abuse the child's sense of security is shattered. The earlier the abuse occurs, the more potentially devastating the impact, since the child may have had no time to develop any secure attachment.[8]

Patients in middle age and older may never have told anyone, including their partner, about the abuse. Since abuse has commonly occurred at the hands of older parental or authority figures victims find it very difficult to trust other authority figures such as doctors. Moreover they will readily experience negative responses (both verbal and non-verbal) from doctors as further abuse.

Inability to trust and form secure relationships with others are common to all survivors of abuse. They will often repeat patterns of victimisation in adult relationships or in the workplace.

> The survivor is left with fundamental problems of basic trust, autonomy and initiative. She approaches the tasks of early adulthood – establishing independence and intimacy – burdened by major impairments in self-care, cognition and memory, in identity and in the capacity to form stable relationships.[8]

Other 'difficult' patients, whilst not having suffered childhood abuse, may well have been victims of emotional trauma in teenage or adult life. Some such patients may have a formal diagnosis of post-traumatic stress disorder, but others may be presenting with physical expression of an underlying emotional trauma.

It follows from this that treatment of the presenting symptoms is unlikely to be successful unless a trusting relationship between patient and caregiver can be established. This is the basis of therapeutic work regardless of the theoretical model of therapy.

ALTERNATIVE MODELS OF CARE

Reductive and Lean models of healthcare do not allow time for unfocused listening. The models encourage directed questioning, and such questioning focuses on the presenting symptoms. Focused questions about abuse are likely to be met with denial and are almost certain be received as abusive themselves. Therapeutic work with survivors of childhood abuse requires the caregiver to enter into the inner world of the patient and sit with them there as a grounding and secure presence. The caregiver must also be aware of his or her own biases and assumptions that he or she brings to the consultation. This where the structured or semi-structured interview fails, in that it is predicated on a series of assumptions. The caregiver who accepts a survivor of childhood abuse as his or her patient must be open to surprise and to the shared pain of the patient. This openness and willingness to share in the patient's experience involves a surrendering of boundaries and a venturing into the transpersonal, which has been well described by Field:[9]

> Even if you throw a rope to a drowning man, it's not help if he can't take hold of it. In certain situations it may be necessary to jump overboard and go to where he happens to be, even though the therapist takes the risk of drowning too. In practice this means that, when a patient is in such a panic he or she cannot even listen, it may be necessary to abandon the defences that separate the therapist and patient, to go down into the patient's desperation, and consciously share it.

The idea of the reparative therapeutic relationship is longstanding:

> … only the actual relationship between analyst and patient as persons could constitute a new reality and thus an indispensable therapeutic factor. Only such a relationship could provide a means of correcting distorted internal relationships and also provide the patient with the opportunity, foreclosed in his childhood, 'to undergo a process of emotional development in the setting of an actual relationship with a reliable and beneficent parental figure'.[10]

Although psychotherapy seems the obvious and easiest way to provide a reparative relationship for survivors of abuse it has been suggested that individuals from a variety of professional backgrounds, as well as some experiences of groups, can be equally effective. What appears to be most important is the pattern of the relationship between patient and caregiver; this has been described as either 'supportive and companionable' or 'dominant versus submissive'. Supportive relating is unthreatening and secure, mutually respectful, protective and exploratory, whereas dominant versus submissive relating involves control and possible coercion from the dominant person and submission from the other.[11]

All too often the patient arriving in the pain clinic relates relationships with other members of the healthcare professions that have been experienced a dominant versus submissive; the traditional doctor/patient relationship has been an unequal and paternalistic one, and although this is changing workloads and lack of personal support may cause the caregiver to fall back onto traditional patterns of relationship.

> Caregivers who are most likely to show D/S [dominant versus submissive] patterns are those whose internal supportive systems undermine their attempts to be competent, whose personal supportive environment cannot be maintained

and who have no effective external support available. When faced with too many careseekers, or ones that are uncooperative, such caregivers feel incompetent and powerless. To regain a sense of control and competence, there is a marked tendency for them to fall back on coercive controlling or avoidant patterns of relating.[12]

The current system of healthcare which favours efficiency (measured in throughput of patients) almost invariably places restraints and limitations on the number, frequency and duration of consultations that can be offered. Such limitation of the caregiver's availability may reinforce the patient's sense of loss and deprivation and perpetuate the cycle of care-seeking. It is arguable that patients will leave the healthcare system of their own accord once their needs are met,[12] but the present situation does not permit testing of this hypothesis. Anecdotal reports have calculated that the cost of intensive, long-term psychotherapy for over 10 years would have been less than the cost of inpatient mental healthcare provided for a victim of childhood abuse.[11]

SUMMARY

A large number of 'difficult' patients referred to the chronic pain clinic have been victims of childhood sexual, emotional or physical abuse. Many have never disclosed this abuse, or have been disbelieved when they attempted disclosure. The current medical model of care offered to these patients is reductive and orientated to efficiency, productivity and rapid throughput.

Victims of childhood abuse have impaired ability to form meaningful relationships with self and others. They readily re-experience the victim role and are likely to become the submissive partner in dominant versus submissive relationships. Healthcare professionals, by virtue of their training and feelings of failure when faced with problems that they cannot readily solve, are equally likely to adopt the dominant role in relationships with these patients. This is experienced by the patient as repetition of a familiar cycle of abuse, combined with feelings of frustration and isolation as yet another person is unable to help them manage their pain.

The opportunity to help victims of childhood abuse is found through a reparative relationship in which there is equality and a willingness to abandon defences and be open to possibilities for learning and growth.

Provision of a reparative relationship is not the sole preserve of the psychotherapist but does require relevant training of selected healthcare professionals. Demonstrating the need for such individuals in the current NHS framework is challenging as management of end-of-the-road chronic pain patients does not lend itself to quantitative randomised controlled trials but rather long-term qualitative case-study research. Assuming that funding becomes available the selection and training of suitable personnel to work with these patients is a little-researched area. Availability of suitably qualified supervisors is limited within the psychotherapy professions, and the concept of supervision is still relatively alien to medical practitioners, but those engaging in this type of work must be offered sufficient support and supervision so that they can work in the intertextual/transpersonal space where healing can occur.

> Only those who will risk going too far can possibly find our how far one can go.
>
> TS Eliot

REFERENCES

1 www.seop.leeds.ac.uk/entries/reduction-biology
2 www.institute.nhs.uk/building_capability/general/lean_thinking.html
3 www.explanatorygap.com/default.aspx
4 www.scribd.com/doc/8981250/Levine-Joseph-Materialism-and-Qualia-The-Explanatory-Gap
5 Clarkson P. *The Therapeutic Relationship.* London and Philadelphia: Whurr; 2003.
6 Green CR, Flowe-Valencia H, Rosenblum L, *et al.* The role of childhood and adulthood abuse among women presenting for chronic pain management. *Clinical Journal of Pain.* 2001; **17**(4): 359–64.
7 Bailey BE, Freedenfeld RN, Sanford Kiser R, *et al.* Lifetime physical and sexual abuse in chronic pain patients: psychosocial correlates and treatment outcomes. *Disability & Rehabilitation.* 2003; **25**(7): 331–42.
8 Fisher G. Existential psychotherapy with adult survivors of sexual abuse. *Journal of Humanistic Psychology.* 2005; **45**(1): 10–40.
9 Field N. *Breakdown and Breakthrough.* London: Routledge; 1996.
10 Fairbairn WRD. On the nature and aims of psychoanalytic treatment. *International Journal of Psychoanalysis.* 1958; **39**: 374–86.
11 McCluskey U, Hooper C-A (eds). *Psychodynamic Perspectives on Abuse.* London: Jessica Kingsley; 2000.
12 Heard D, Lake B. *The Challenge of Attachment for Care-Giving.* London: Routledge; 1997.

FURTHER READING

➤ Moi T (ed). *The Kristeva Reader.* Columbia: Columbia University Press; 1986.
➤ Rowan J, Jacobs M. *The Therapist's Use of the Self.* Maidenhead: Open University Press; 2002.
➤ Spinelli E. *Demystifying Therapy.* Ross-on-Wye: PCCS Books; 2006.
➤ Spinelli E. *Tales of Un-knowing: Therapeutic Encounters from an Existential Perspective.* Ross-on-Wye: PCCS Books; 2006.

CHAPTER 7

Exploiting the placebo response: culpable deception or a neglected path in the search for healing?

Peter Wemyss-Gorman

The placebo response is a fascinating subject which seems to go to the heart of the mysterious relationships between mind, brain and body – Patrick Wall indeed considered it to be at the heart of understanding pain.[1] The main purpose of this chapter is to explore the ethical dilemmas that can arise from pain and in particular the ethical aspects of deliberately exploiting it. It may, however, be helpful to those not familiar with the literature first to survey some of the background.

The term placebo is said to be derived from '*Placebo dominum in regione Dominum*' ('I will please the lord in the land of the living'), the opening words of the Vespers for the dead. In mediaeval France 'Placebo singers' were sometimes people unconnected with the deceased who came to a funeral in the hope of getting free food and drink, and the term came to imply simulators of grief or flatterers. Later the word 'placebo' seems to have acquired connotations of pleasing someone by telling them want they expect or want to hear, and came into medical parlance, mainly pertaining to quackery, at the beginning of the 18th century

There have been several attempts to replace the term with something with more intrinsic meaning, such as 'context effect' or 'meaning response', but as it has the virtues of both brevity and universal recognition I shall continue to use placebo in this chapter. It has been argued[2] that placebo *response* is a better expression than the more widely used placebo *effect*, as of course placebos defined as inert substances can by definition have no *pharmacological* effect whatever. They do, however, evoke a response in the person receiving them, which may have the *effect of relieving a symptom*; this may not be the direct effect of the placebo but is the consequence of giving it. This may seem to be labouring an apparently semantic point, but it illustrates the difficulty of making definitive statements about placebos when our understating of how they work is so incomplete. The word 'nocebo' has been coined for the opposite effect to placebo, where the expectation is that a treatment will not work and reduces its efficacy.

WHAT ARE PLACEBOS?

To describe a placebo as a pharmacologically inert substance is easy enough, but comprehensive definition of the placebo *effect* (or response) which applies in all circumstances has always been elusive. It seems to have become even more difficult to find as we have acquired deeper understanding of the consequences of giving placebos. It may indeed be simpler to identify what placebos are *not* and do *not* do than what they are. To begin with, the placebo response is not a 'purely' psychological, cognitive phenomenon. Although subjective symptoms such as pain and depression seem to be the most amenable to relief by placebos, objective 'physical' symptoms such as swelling of the jaw after tooth extraction have been shown to be reduced by placebo,[3] and they are effective in conditions such as asthma with objective clinical manifestations. Patients with obstructive cardiomyopathy whose pacemakers were switched off without their knowledge not only continued to experience fewer symptoms, but the thickening of their heart muscle was also reduced.[4] A placebo was shown to raise dopamine levels in the brains of patients with Parkinson's disease.[5]

MISCONCEPTIONS

There are several common misconceptions about placebos.[1,2] Among them, one thankfully no longer widely held is the suggestion that they can differentiate between organic and mental disease or 'hysteria', and that pain relieved by them is not 'real' (dismissed by Wall as 'cruel and dangerous nonsense which flies in the face of overwhelming evidence to the contrary'[1]). Placebo responders have been thought to conform to a special mentality or personality type but there is no evidence for this, although it probably is true that there may be a somewhat greater placebo response in neurotic, anxious or dependent subjects. There is a common belief dating back to a misreading of Beecher's classic studies in the 1950s that there is a fixed proportion of patients who respond to placebo, usually quoted as 30%, but the actual range is from 0 to nearly 100%. Intuition (which might betray our enduring dualistic mindset) might seem to lead to the assumption that placebos would only modify the affective dimensions of pain such as unpleasantness, but there is evidence that they can reduce the actual intensity of pain.

But the most important realisation in our present context is that the assumption underlying both the concept of placebo-controlled trials and traditional attitudes to deliberate placebo prescription that placebos are the equivalent of no therapy is demonstrably false. Pharmacologically effective drugs have powerful placebo effects of their own. Even as potent a drug as morphine has been shown to be much more effective in patients identified as strong placebo responders than in non-responders. The effect of expectation has been difficult to quantify but is clearly considerable and may even sometimes exceed specific effect. Placebo-controlled trials with a 'no-intervention' comparison show clear evidence of a big placebo effect on the pain of osteoarthritis. The effect size is about 0.6, whereas for all other interventions it is about 0.2. So in this situation placebos are apparently three times more powerful.[6] The effect of any drug or intervention is always the result of a complex interaction between positive and negative specific and context effects, and the two are almost impossible to separate or quantify relative to one another.

HOW DO THEY 'WORK'?

The search for a biological substrate for the analgesic effect of placebos seemed to take a major step forward in 1978 with the Levine's observation that naloxone, an opioid antagonist, reversed placebo analgesia, suggesting that endogenous opioid mechanisms were involved.[7] This has been confirmed by more recent studies of opioid receptors. These findings might seem to be supported by positron emission tomography (PET) which demonstrates that placebo analgesia is accompanied by activation of the same brain regions as when an analgesic drug is given,[8] and functional magnetic resonance imaging (fMRI) which showed reduced activity after placebo in pain-sensitive brain areas.[9] (Functional brain imaging shows *where* task-related activity occurs in the brain. This of course is not the same as showing *how* psychological mechanisms function, and, like *neuropsychology* and *neurophysiology, functional imaging* is only one window of understanding into the function of the brain and its relation to mind.) There is evidence that intact and functioning prefrontal areas are necessary for a placebo response to pain and this may be lost in advanced Alzheimer's disease.[10] Although neurobiology is as yet a long way from providing all the answers, perhaps its most useful contribution to the debate has been to help change the perception of placebo as something rather nebulous and the stuff of psychobabble, to that of a 'real' phenomenon worthy of serious scientific scrutiny. There has been a tendency in the past among researchers to regard the placebo response only as a confounding factor in clinical trials and an unmitigated nuisance, but more recently there has been some rapprochement between researchers and clinicians who have long recognised its therapeutic potential.

The main psychological mechanisms thought to underlie the placebo response are expectation and conditioning. (Conditioning as in the classical experiments of Pavlov and his dogs whose salivation with the offer of food and the simultaneous ringing of a bell could after some repetition be induced by the bell alone.) Relief of anxiety may also be involved on occasion but clearly does not provide a complete explanation. It seems fairly self-evident that the expectation or belief that a treatment will or will not work will affect its outcome, and this intuition has been backed up by many studies. Factors influencing expectation include the presentation (including the colour) of a pill, the impressiveness of an interventional gadget and (most significantly in the context of this chapter) the impression given by the doctor* of confidence, authority, etc. and the rapport between patient and doctor. There is good experimental evidence that conditioning mechanisms are also involved in the human placebo response, especially with regard to its magnitude.[1] Wall has proposed that the placebo is not a stimulus but an appropriate response to pain defined as a 'need state', like hunger, which can be terminated by appropriate, 'consummatory' action.[1] Moerman and Jonas[11] have argued that the thing which makes a placebo more or less effective (and enhances or detracts from the effect of any medical intervention) is the *meaning* it holds for the recipient (e.g. red tablets are seen as stimulants and blue ones as depressants) and that the term placebo should be replaced by 'meaning response'. One intriguing suggestion is that the placebo response derives from our evolution as animists. Our ancient forbears believed that everything in the natural world was animated and had power over them, which explained things that happened to them like fire, flood and illness. The belief that power comes from outside inwards has persisted as part of our psychology. So the modern pill is the equivalent of the shaman's incantations and amulets, and the placebo response an unconscious expression of an atavistic belief in magic (M Kell, personal communication). Another less well-known theory postulates that context can evoke the 'nurturing response'. As animals evolved into social groups and the maternal instinct developed, the primitive 'shut down' and 'fight or flight' responses to threat became supplemented by the instinct to protect and nurture other individuals, and to respond to this. We learn in infancy to respond to stress or pain by 'shut down' or 'fight or flight'. This may persist to adulthood but can be modified by the nurturing response, and if the healer evokes this by making us feel safe we will be less distressed, and the effect of intervention enhanced (P Dieppe,

---

* There are many professionals – nurses, physiotherapists and psychologists and others as well as physicians – who practice in pain management. For the sake avoiding a more cumbersome term I have used 'doctor' throughout this chapter but in many cases this can be read as shorthand for 'health professional'. And I make no apologies for using the male gender inclusively.

personal communication). (Porges maintains that this involves the midbrain, the autonomic nervous system and specifically the vagus nerves, and has elaborated this into his polyvagal theory.[12])

So much then for a quick gallop through the background except for pausing for a moment to consider the question – do placebos 'work' at all? The false impression of a placebo effect (or for that matter a 'true' therapeutic effect) is sometimes obtained by neglecting the natural history of a condition, for instance, where episodes of a relapsing condition are going to get better any-way. A major meta-analysis published in the *New England Journal of Medicine* in 2001[13] set off a storm of controversy by seeming to suggest, if not prove, that placebos have no effect whatever, at least in the setting of clinical trials. There did, however, seem to be an exception in the case of pain and the conclusion of the debate seemed to be that most people accepted that they do 'work', at least some of the time in some people.

MIND-BODY MEDICINE

We have rightly rejected the dualistic view of pain as either in the body or the mind when it comes to diagnosis but have we really embraced the positive therapeutic potential of mind-body interaction? Should 'mind-body medicine' be brought back from the fringes of alternative medicine? Unfortunately much of the literature on the latter seems to contain enough pseudo-science mixed with the 'real' science to raise the sceptical hackles of most scientifically trained doctors. But the vast amount of research that has gone into elucidating the neurobiological mechanisms of pain perception and the like has been persistently disappointing in terms of therapeutic spin-off and might even be suspected of having led us into a blind alley. Might mind-body interaction point us to one possible way through this therapeutic impasse? There has indeed been some work on this,[14] particularly in the context of placebo, but it seems minuscule in volume compared with 'biomedical' research, and much of it is from a predominantly psychological perspective. Although the mind-body concept pervades the whole of medicine, I think it could be reasonably claimed that pain therapists and researchers have led the way in this direction. It will no doubt be contended that getting research handles on such an apparently nebulous subject is extremely difficult and obtaining funding probably even more so. If Pat Wall believed that placebos are at the heart of the understanding of pain I hope he might not have entirely disagreed with the above. But this is a speculative diversion, and we need to get back to the practical and ethical aspects of placebo.

ETHICAL PROBLEMS

In research

Randomised, placebo-controlled trials have long been considered the gold standard for evaluating new drugs and interventions. The extensive literature on the technical aspects of placebos in research is of limited concern to the general reader (the reviews by McQuay and Moore (2005)[2] and Reynolds (2000)[15] are suggested for those interested) but a few examples will illustrate the sort of problems clinical researchers face in the use of placebos. First, where the placebo response is high, as in the case of analgesics, placebo-controlled trials may be of little value. Secondly, they cannot be justified when withholding active treatment could cause serious harm to a patient. Indeed it may be argued that it is always unethical to give a placebo where an effective treatment exists. But comparative trials, where the new drug is compared with an existing one, may expose more patients to harm because if the difference between the drugs is small a larger number of subjects must take part. (Comparative trials are a particular problem for drug companies: a company, having invested several years and several million pounds in developing a new drug, will be reluctant to compare it with a competitor or generic product unless it is absolutely sure that its product is superior. Companies do not want to take the risk of finding that their drug may actually be inferior to, or no better but more expensive than, the other.). A wide consensus has evolved that there is no ethical objection to the use of placebos in trials where no significant or irreversible harm can ensue from withholding active treatment (e.g. in conditions such as baldness which is frequently not treated at all) or where no effective treatment for a condition exists. Where an effective treatment does already exist there must be a compelling reason for including a placebo arm and there must be scrupulous precautions to minimise the possibility of harm. There might appear to be a conflict between the rights and interests of the patients involved in studies and the objective demands of science, but trials that cannot produce reliable conclusions are in themselves unethical.

In clinical practice

In contrast to the extensive literature on ethical aspects of clinical research, much of it only of great interest to researchers, considerably less has been written on the use of placebo in everyday practice,[16] although this might appear to be of much wider importance, especially to those outside the medical profession. Perhaps this is because it is perceived to be an academic or even esoteric matter as few modern doctors would even dream of prescribing a treatment they know to be useless and lying about it. But I would doubt if there are many who would not agree that placebos can be powerful therapeutic weapons, which with a few exceptions were of course the only ones available to our medical forefathers up to barely a couple of generations ago. Physicians from Hippocrates up to the present era of scientific, evidence-based medicine have advocated the benefits of 'benevolent deception'.[17] The attitude of the Hippocratic physician to his patient was paternalistic, and truthfulness either about diagnosis or treatment was not considered necessary or even desirable. It was explicitly recognised that a cure was often effected only by virtue of the patient's faith in the physician, who was encouraged to exploit his position of authority as the possessor of esoteric knowledge. Hippocratic principles continued to dominate medicine right up to the Renaissance, and even in the 17th century when doctors were identifying and studying specific diseases (and anatomy), there still seems to have been no attempt to distinguish placebos from specific remedies. Deception which seemed to be in the patient's interest continued to be acceptable without question even as late as the end of the 18th century. With the emergence of modern medical ethics at the beginning of the 19th century (notably in the writings of Thomas Percival) there was much debate on the propriety of using placebos which by then had been clearly identified, but benevolent deception continued to be generally regarded as an essential skill of the physician.

It was indeed only in the last century that attitudes to placebos began to change diametrically. Although there remained relatively few powerful pharmacological agents with specific effects on specific conditions for much of the first half of the century, anything which could not be so described came to be regarded as of little value. The enormous advances in pharmacology in the last 50 years have not only consolidated this view but apparently removed any pretext for deliberately using placebos. Their use as controls in clinical trials has until relatively recently been predicated on the assumption that they are completely inert. These perceptions, along with the consensus that patients must be involved in decisions about their own treatment and kept fully informed about every aspect of this and their condition, had all but banished the concept of benevolent deceit , and with it placebo therapy, to history. The ethical position seemed simple and incontrovertible: deliberate placebo therapy, along with every other form of quackery and dishonesty, had no place whatever in modern medicine.

However, deepening understanding of the power and modes of action of placebo has brought the suspicion that the position may not be as cut and dried as this. There seems to be some dissociation between the philosophical arguments and a pragmatic approach to clinical practice. The former are traditionally concerned mainly with the issue of deception. Deception, lying and dishonesty are generally regarded as unacceptable in any from of human relationship, and especially so in the case of the doctor/patient relationship, based as it is on trust. (A case can possibly be made out that patients who want their doctor to behave paternalistically trust him to prescribe whatever he deems good for them, so deceit is not a breach of that trust. But at best this is of limited general application.) Against this is the utilitarian position of the importance of the consequences of actions. If deceiving a patient is in his best interests or brutal honesty is likely to cause distress (as in the giving of bad prognostic news without any attempt to preserve some hope), it may be not only justifiable but obligatory to be economical with the truth. These considerations might be seen to apply in a fairly straightforward way to the actual prescription of a sugar pill in the guise of an effective drug. Situations where a doctor can find a pretext for deliberately prescribing a treatment which he knows to be completely devoid of direct effect are rare. It has, however, been suggested that there is no ethical objection to prescribing a sugar pill if you tell the patient what it is.[18] This might seem to detract somewhat from its possible efficacy, but it has been contended that revealing to patients how well they have responded to placebo and educating them regarding the positive effects of expectation might enhance the efficacy of both placebo and active treatments.[19]

A possible case for utilising measures without established direct therapeutic effects could be made with regard to 'alternative' therapies, notably homeopathy. Although few doctors would actually prescribe these there are probably not many who would actively dissuade their patients from seeking help from alternative practitioners. Many of these seem particularly adept at exploiting and manipulating the placebo effect without conscious deception because they believe in their own remedies. (The question of whether homeopathy really just might possibly have specific effects is fascinating and demands a completely unfamiliar way of looking at scientific evidence, but is not relevant to our present argument.) To this day, in many parts of the world the lack of resources for modern Western medicine obliges people to resort to traditional healing which largely relies on faith in it in a scientifically unsophisticated population. This seems often to be very effective and a great deal better that nothing. And for that matter how much does Western medicine rely on an arguably misplaced faith in science?

EXPECTATION IN PAIN MEDICINE

The position in pain medicine is rather more complicated and nuanced. Although few practitioners would ever consider deliberately prescribing an inert 'remedy' and trying to deceive the patient into believing in its potency, the temptation – some would say the justification – to use a therapy which seems to help some people but whose efficacy has never been irrefutably proved, and indeed one harbours some doubts about, occurs almost daily. This is a particular problem in chronic pain therapy: patients usually end up in pain clinics when all well-recognised and tested means of alleviating their pain have failed. To take the very common problem of low back pain as an example, patients may have had every known analgesic, at least one failed operation and much else. It may be in their best interests to tell them frankly that there is no known cure for their problem and concentrate on helping them to live with their pain. There are, however, a number of procedures that have become the province of pain doctors which may provide temporary and occasionally prolonged relief. These include injecting local anaesthetics and steroids into the facet joints of the spine, and disrupting the function of the nerves supplying them. For various reasons it has been very difficult to construct objective clinical trials to establish the 'true' value of these treatments, but their use has been long justified by the accumulation of anecdotal evidence in the experience of individual doctors. Their place in the management of chronic low back pain has been a contentious matter among pain doctors with some proponents and opponents adopting polarised positions. The majority are probably trying to find a compromise (as described by Ian Yellowlees elsewhere in Chapter 5). But even the most enthusiastic interventionists would have to admit that failure to help very much in the long run is more common than one might have hoped. The same applies in varying measures to the use of many drugs, for instance, those used in neuropathic pain; although trials of these are easier to construct success rates are rarely as high as might be wished. But we all too often have nothing better to offer to desperate patients.

As mentioned earlier, all therapeutic agents and interventions, at least in the context of pain, depend in some measure for their potency on the placebo response and the effect of expectation. So is strict and objective honesty always morally superior to trying to enhance the power of interventions by increasing patients' expectations of success and not being entirely frank about the possibility of failure? In practice it is actually quite difficult *not* to use the placebo response, even unconsciously. Patients desperate for relief desperately want their treatment to work, and the doctor, if he has any humanity, is equally anxious to help. Unless he goes out of his way to stress the possibility of failure (and thereby probably provoking a negative, nocebo response) the patient will assume that he believes in the treatments he is offering – and the doctor is highly motivated to believe in them himself despite paucity of objective evidence for their efficacy. But if he had the objectivity of a computer would he be a better doctor?

CONCLUSION: A PERSONAL DILEMMA

To conclude on a more personal level: I suppose I never gave the matter much thought until taken to task many years ago by a young colleague for failing to 'sell' treatments more positively. I tried feebly to defend myself but have remained in some ambivalence about the subject ever since. Why was I somewhat diffident in the way I presented treatments? I do not dispute the value of a good rapport with patients, being seen to be interested in them and their complaints, having a confident and reasonably authoritative manner and so on, not only in themselves but as part of the therapeutic process. But I have always felt a compulsion to at least try to be as honest as possible, influenced perhaps not so much by ethical scruples as by my reaction to the sad stories angry and disillusioned patients told me about Mr X and Dr Y who had assured them with irresistible confidence that their wonderful (and sometimes very expensive) operation or intervention was bound to cure their pain, and when it failed they were made to feel that it was their own fault, or that their continuing unabated symptoms were 'not genuine'. (I should perhaps hesitate to label such an approach as quackery as of course these things do work sometimes, but I do occasionally wonder if some of these people are not the modern equivalent of the quacks of yesteryear, with the essential difference that their 'remedies' have much more potential for harm than coloured pills and nasty tasting potions.) So I think people who have learnt to distrust doctors do appreciate honesty, and anyway many will probably have irretrievably lost the expectation of benefit which is a major component of the placebo response.

Looking back, I often wonder if I should have 'sold' my interventions more confidently, and without in the back of my mind thinking about what I would say to patients when they returned no better. Indeed towards the end of my career I seemed to be doing fewer and fewer interventions, not as a matter of policy but because more and more patients declined my offer of one, probably because they perceived that I was not very sure if it would help them or not. Had I done them a disservice? On the other hand, if I too failed to help them despite my assurances, would they not be even more disillusioned and depressed? No doubt this is something that every clinician has to work out for himself, and I hope that many have done this more successfully than I suspect I ever did. What I did try to do was to give people justifiable hope rather than unrealistic expectations, remembering always that many probably had an indefinite future of living with pain to look forward to, and that I was trying to lay the foundations of what might well become a long and difficult therapeutic relationship.

REFERENCES

1 Wall PD. The placebo and the placebo response. In: Melzack R, Wall PD. *Textbook of Pain*. 4th ed. Edinburgh: Churchill Livingstone; 1999. pp. 1419–30.
2 McQuay HJ, Moore RA. Placebo. *Postgraduate Medical Journal*. 2005; **81**: 155–60.
3 Ho KH, Hashish I, Salmon P, *et al*. Reduction of postoperative swelling by a placebo effect. *Journal of Psychosomatic Research*. 1988; **32**(2): 197–205.
4 Linde C, Gadler F, Kappenbuger L, *et al*. Placebo effect of pacemaker implantation in obstructive cardiomyopathy. *Am J Cardiol*. 1999; **83**(2): 903–7.
5 De la Fuente-Fernadez R, Stoessl AJ. The placebo effect in Parkinson's disease. *Trends in Neurosciences*. 2002; **25**(6): 302–6.

6 Zhang W, Robertson J, Jones AC, *et al.* The placebo effect and its determinants in osteoarthritis: meta-analysis of randomised controlled trials. *Annals of Rheumatic Diseases.* 2008; **67**: 1716–23.

7 Levine JD, Gordon NC, Fields HL. The mechanism of placebo analgesia. *Lancet.* 1978; **2**: 654–7.

8 Petrovic P, Kalso E, Peterson KM, *et al.* Placebo and opioid analgesia – imaging a shared neuronal network. *Science.* 2002; **295**: 1737–40.

9 Wager TD, Rilling JK, Smith EE, *et al.* Placebo-induced changes in fMRI in the anticipation and experience of pain. *Science.* 2004; **303**(5661): 1162–7.

10 Benedetti F, Mayberg HS, Wager TD, *et al.* Loss of expectation-related mechanisms in Alzheimer's disease makes analgesic therapies less effective. *Pain.* 2006; **121**(1): 133–44.

11 Moerman DB, Jonas WB. Deconstructing the placebo effect and finding the meaning response. *Annals of Internal Medicine.* 2002; **136**(6): 471–6.

12 Porges S, Orienting in a defensive world: mammalian modifications of our evolutionary heritage. A polyvagal theory. *Psychophysiology.* 1995; **32**: 301–18.

13 Hrobartsson A, Gotzche PC. Is the placebo effect powerless? An analysis of clinical trials compared with no-treatment. *New England Journal of Medicine.* 2001; **344**: 1594–1602.

14 Astin JA, Shapiro SL, Eisenberg DM, *et al.* Mind-body medicine: state of the science, implications for practice. *The Journal of the American Board of Family Practice.* 2003; **16**: 131–47.

15 Reynolds T. The ethics of placebo-controlled trials. *Annals of Internal Medicine.* 2000; **133**(6): 491–2.

16 Biller-Adorno N. The use of the placebo effect in clinical medicine – ethical blunder or ethical imperative? *Science and Engineering Ethics.* 2004; **10**: 43–50.

17 Rawlinson MC. Truth-telling and paternalism in the clinic: philosophical reflections on the use of placebos in medical practice. In: White L, Tursky B, Schwartz GE, *et al* (eds). *Placebo: Theory and Mechanisms.* New York: Guildford Press; 1985. pp. 403–19.

18 Brody H. The lie that heals: the ethics of giving placebos. *Annals of Internal Medicine.* 1982; **97**: 112–18.

19 Keefe F, Abernethy AP, Affleck G. Don't ask, don't tell? Revealing placebo responses to research participants and patients. *Pain.* 2008; **135**(3): 213–14.

FURTHER READING

➤ Fabrizio B. *Placebo Effects: understanding the mechanisms in health and disease.* Oxford: Oxford University Press; 2008.

➤ Fields HL, Price DD. Placebo analgesia. In: McMahon SB, Koltzenburg M (eds). *Wall and Melzack's Textbook of Pain.* 5th ed. Edinburgh: Elsevier Churchill-Livingstone; 2005. pp. 361–7.

➤ Wikipedia. *Placebo.* http://en.wikipedia.org/wiki/Placebo (accessed 5 May 2011).

CHAPTER 8

Prostituting pain

Kate Maguire

Pain has occupied me since I was a very young child, not because I had experienced any particularly severe physical pain, only the odd toothache and tonsillitis towards which I demonstrated the usual human capacity for adaptive behaviour and healing, but for two other, very important reasons. Firstly, my father had a book in which there were pictures of the Holocaust. They have haunted me all my life, reinforced by my work in and among people in conflict zones where that other human capacity, to inflict pain, thrives. Secondly, while the dentist could solve the toothache and the doctor the tonsillitis, there seemed to be no cure for a child's feelings of perplexity, of having landed on the wrong planet, of unworthiness, feelings that I could not utter, could not find words for, could not even identify as pain but which clung onto me as pervasively and tenaciously as Maupassant's Horla,[1] threatening to drag me wordless down into the depths of despair.

These, and I am sure other influences, led me to become a political anthropologist of that perennial area of pain, the Middle East. I believe anthropology taught me more about human relational behaviour than psychology did. It taught me about humankind's relationship to the world; about non-judgemental acceptance of the other; about universal types to whom we can find a connection no matter how alien the culture seems to be to us; about the art of language which can communicate complex concepts and experiences in simple images and about a deep respect for the spiritual not as a separate entity, a religious trick, a neurosis but an essential part of the health of the individual and the group. Perhaps it was Levi-Strauss's definition of anthropology which really won me over. It was, of course, the 1960s.

> Anthropology will never succeed in being a dispassionate science like astronomy which springs from the contemplation of things at a distance. It is the outcome of a historical process which has made the larger part of mankind subservient to the other. During this process millions of innocent human beings have had

their resources plundered and their institutions and beliefs destroyed whilst they themselves were ruthlessly killed, thrown into bondage and contaminated by diseases they were unable to resist. Anthropology is daughter to this era of violence. Its capacity to assess more objectively the facts pertaining to the human condition appropriately reflects, on the epistemological level, a state of affairs in which one part of mankind treated the other as an object.[2]

Getting to grips with the systemic principles and cultural variances of power and powerlessness, while intellectually satisfying, was of absolutely no use when confronted with dead and dying bodies in the streets and refugee camps of a war-torn Beirut, so I decided to retrain as a psychotherapist working with survivors of torture and extreme experiences looking for ways to bridge the gap between the feeling and the word, a kind of Hermetic quest to connect two very different realms of experience: those in extreme pain and those not. I have always liked the notion of psychotherapists being of the Hermetic tradition, not he of the winged feet but of the older Hermes Trismegistus of the Alexandrians. They derived this complex and intriguing figure from their predecessors, the ancient Egyptians, who, in their wisdom, had recognised that as there was so obviously a deep chasm of understanding between the realms of the mortals and the gods, it would require a skilled interlocutor, a god in fact, to bridge it. So they embodied this role in Thoth, Three Times Great, hence Hermes Trismegistus. Many ancient civilisations have awarded the status of god to the concept of connection. This god is always a trickster, a story teller, a humorist, full of human foibles, behaving just a little like a god, very human indeed then. Not that psychotherapists are gods, only that they are, at their best, connectors between different parts of the human being which have become split off; between one human being and another and between different realms of experience. This is not always successfully achieved through words as people in severe pain, psychological and/or physical, are often wary of words. Ordinary words can not only fail to bridge the gap, but can in fact actively contribute to it.

> … for the person in pain, so incontestably and unnegotiably present in it that 'having pain' may come to be thought of as the most vibrant example of what it is to 'have certainty', while for the other person it is so elusive that 'hearing about pain' may exist as the primary model for what it is 'to have doubt'. Thus pain becomes unsharably into our midst as at once that which cannot be denied and that which cannot be confirmed.[3]

A few years ago I had the opportunity to spend time in different pain units in London doing research on the language and concepts of pain. The following two encounters may illustrate where I am coming from in trying to grapple with the concepts and appropriate treatments for a range of deep pains which are physiologically and psychologically bound together. I have altered some of the details to protect the identity of the patients.*

Mary

Mary came in to see the doctor with severe pain in her shoulder. She had been coming to his clinic for years and before him to the previous consultant. She was possibly in her 70s but her dress and make-up were more those of a teenager of another time down to the short skirt and bows in her shoes and hair, even younger – a kind of Shirley Temple. She was charming and disappeared behind a curtain with the consultant whom I could hear saying that he really couldn't give her any more cortisone. She was flirting beautifully with him, confident that she would eventually get her way. I sat with her husband, a dapper man who was obviously still very much in love with his wife. They had never had children. I asked him how he was and how he was coping. He was very surprised at my enquiry saying no one had ever asked him this before. He said it wasn't easy because sometimes his wife was fine and at others time the pain was shocking. Did he know what caused it? No. It had just come upon her in her 20s and no one could find a source. He hoped the doctor would be kind enough to give her something as they had a wedding to go to. Had they been coming to this hospital for long? Oh yes, they had lost a baby here just after the war and had been coming back ever since. He thought it was her way to be close to the baby she never got to take home, the pain relief was like her taking her baby home instead of leaving the baby here and taking her pain home. Had he ever mentioned this to his wife, to the doctors. No never.

Faris

There were two students and myself sitting in. The consultant is a well-known and respected pain practitioner. His students were obviously in awe of him. A man in his 30s came in complaining of severe pain in his back. His English was not fluent. The consultant asked the students

(continued)

---

* In this text I mostly use the word 'patient' for convenience although psychotherapists mostly use 'client'. This can vary depending on the setting especially for those working in medical settings.

to take a careful history while he went to attend to an emergency and to consult me if they encountered any problems. The man said he had had this pain since he was tortured in his country, an Arab country. He couldn't sleep. It was driving him crazy. The man looked sleep deprived, haunted even. The students asked if he had family. Yes, he said, a son and now a new baby girl. The students were reluctant to proceed much beyond the standard checklist because his English was not fluent enough either to understand fully their questions or to give an answer and he was becoming very agitated. The students decided quite reasonably that he would need a scan and definitely pain medication. I decided to chat to him in Arabic while we waited for the consultant to return. He seemed very relieved. I asked him how long he had had the pain. He said over 10 years. Why did he think it was worse now, needing the attention of the doctor? It is not worse. It is the same. But I can't sleep, I can't sleep. Because of the pain? No, because of the baby, it won't stop crying during the night, for weeks, it is driving me mad. I need to take something to sleep or I'm afraid I will kill my child. Please give me something to help me not kill my child.

There are many reasons why we do not ask certain questions, not least because we are afraid of what it will open up and then what will we do, who will we send them to, where are the resources? Is it not better to provide pain relief and then the other things will sort themselves out? Yes, we know pain relief does not always work but what else can be done? I am not on a soap box here advocating psychotherapy. What I would like to do is share some ideas with you about the language, concepts and treatment of pain, extreme pain. What we all have in common as psychotherapists is that we work with pain, all kinds of pain but mostly existential pain. Pain is a fact of life. Even if we succeed in finding a total biopain reliever we are still left with existential/psychosocial pain unless we are happy to be drugged for the rest of our lives. Although pain is our job, many of us are often unprepared for what we hear or perhaps prepared too well to the extent that we have our clinical defence techniques of detachment and objectifying which perhaps serve the purpose of not rendering ourselves powerless with the patient or with the world. We cannot afford to identify too much with the patient in case we can see connections to our own lives and thoughts or begin to feel guilty at our social or political passivity. So what do we do when a level of pain comes through the door which is out of normal experience, intensely challenging and disempowering and even traumatising for the listener, a level of pain say in the form of S. We read the notes. He has attempted suicide four times. His wife is trying to get an injunction to keep him away from her and their two children because he is sick. He had seen his father blown up by a land mine in front of him while they were in the rice fields when he was about four then he was taken prisoner for several months by the Khmer Rouge when he was only 11. Do we offer cognitive behavioural techniques for PTSD? EMDR (eye movement desensitisation and reprocessing)? Do we refer on to a hard-pressed refugee agency? Do we send him back to the GP? Do we talk to the psychiatrist about pain relief and antidepressants? Do we calculate that six sessions might not help him much but it would be the 'right' thing to do and anyway it is all that can be afforded? Do we find ourselves saying that our particular approach is not appropriate and he would need to see someone else? Should we put him on the waiting list so we can think about it later? Let us move a little closer to S.

An extract from some of S's writing before a session:

> I don't want to hear that I am the one who hurts or harms anyone because I only harm myself whenever I see those bad tortures in the camps of the Khmer Rouge …

> I want to swallow my children, both of them, keep them inside me and carry them everywhere I go, so there is no one who can come and give them any problems. Also they both won't lose the love they want to have and no one will come to do the torturing to them.

> The beautiful dream has gone and there is less meaning to hope. Love has more pain to love, the world has become too small to walk … one day I will find a space to stand on in this wide world and things will change for me … if there is someone who can see me as a person. I would ask her to be my friend a good friend only because I have no more love to give to anyone.

And what do we do as a doctor, a psychiatrist, a psychologist/therapist, a social worker, a human being when a Pedro comes through the door …

PEDRO OR THE DEMOLITION

> There comes a moment (moment in a structural sense) where the pain moves away from the aggression to the physical body of the subject towards the more destructive experience of dereliction. This moment occurs after a time of imprisonment and torture which varies according to the individual and the context of the situation. It can be a few hours, a few days, a few months.

> Starting with the intensity of the physical pain, sensory deprivation, obscurity, blindfolding, the breaking of all affective and effective links of the personal world

which was loved, the subject finally arrives at the constant presence of the painful body, hurting, broken, totally at the mercy of the torturer; all other perceptions of the world, which are not centred on the present experiences, cease to exist. We call this moment: **the demolition.**[4]

In these two examples there is the interweaving of extreme physical, emotional and existential pain which, in many, defies words and sets the survivor down on an abandoned rock of pain, like Philoctetes, cast onto a small island by his companions at the onset of the Trojan War because they could not bear to hear or smell his pain:

Alone on this inhospitable shore,
Where waves forever beat and tempests roar,
How could he e'er hope or comfort know,
Or painful life support beneath such weight of woe.[5]

This island can be several thousand miles away from the practitioner's, from most people's, in fact, so far that a connection to the mainland needs an informed interlocutor.

It's not that I cannot explain that you won't understand, it's that you won't understand that I cannot explain.[6]

One encounter while supervising was a salutary lesson in not taking at face value that a patient's ability to talk about his or her experiences was an indication of good mental health, of a reconnection to the separated parts and to the world. I believe it so important that I have used his words for the title of this chapter. A survivor of torture related quite fluently to the therapist an account of his torture. The therapist remarked on his ability to do this. He responded that of course he could do this. He had to do this. It was the only way he could get into this country and ensure his wife and children were safe, it being a prerequisite of entry and the guaranteed assurance of a secure roof and some benefits until he got better. The therapist responded that she understood – no he said, you don't understand – I have been prostituting my pain. This patient had become plagued with headaches and dissociated from his experiences so what he talked about and his felt experience had become split off from and distrustful of each other creating a tension which was pushing him to the edge of trauma-induced psychosis.

Words for such levels of pain which are associated with torture, and by torture I also include childhood abuse and deprivation and any actions which are on the far fringes of normal experience, can never portray the total physiological and psychological devastation of the experience. As such, words can appear to be the spokesperson for the cognitive, the rationalising, detached, sensible, pull-yourself-together, parental voice that betrays the emotional part of that individual regressed to a child, shamed, stripped of any defence, of any comfort, of any security, of any sense of trust in human beings, by the infliction of torture. Torture is the ultimate betrayal of humanity, the irreversible stripping away of the mask of illusion of 'civilisation'. It is this voice that needs to be heard without overwhelming the other.

There is a growing number of research studies into pain in neuroscience and neurobiology giving greater understanding of how the brain functions in relation to pain. These findings also give a scientific validation to the clinical evidence practitioners have gathered over several years of practice and therefore come as no surprise. Some of these were discussed in a report in *The Times* in 2008[7] with the main conclusions emphasising the interlink between physiological and psychological pain; the recognition of the psychological being as important as the physiological; responses to pain being individual; and the pain of trauma enduring beyond the healing of the physiological pain.

These findings may add to the library of information about how the brain or individual brains process pain and the eventual development of more tailor-made interventions but the relevance to the issue of torture and extreme experiences is not so clear. There is no doubt and never has been that in torture the link between the physical and the emotional is irrefutable. It is the aim of torture to dismantle the total functioning of a human being through fear of and infliction of extreme physical and emotional pain. Systematic torture is designed on a deprivation of needs scale as in the Maslow hierarchy which is discussed below (*see* Figure 8.1 and Maslow's hierarchy of needs on page 105). In torture, the mind and body can become spilt and separated and mistrustful of each other. When the mind wants to die a prison doctor or the skills of the torturer can keep the body alive; when the body wants to die the mind makes it go on living. The body becomes a vehicle of pain to which the mind can no longer relate. For torture and extreme experiences survivors, it is not about how much pain you feel, but what influences survival, how the fragmented or split parts of a person's being can be glued back together and what the nature and dynamics of survival are which are more than biologically defined.

If we go back to the Hermetic notion, the great strength of this embodied concept is the ability of Hermes to tell stories, to trick the brain into understanding, to mediate the cognitive and the emotional, to encourage two voices to speak at the same time and to be eventually attuned to each other and, once again, to the world. The language of Hermes Trismegistus was metaphor. Metaphor sits well between the cognitive and the creative brain. It is open to reasoning but is not logical, it is creative yet grammatically sound defying the boundaries of words and action. It is subjective and objective at the same time, local and universal, short in words but gives access to an astonishingly large data base of meaning and information across time and cultures. It is not unlike Einstein's $E = mc^2$, a few symbols which represent the distillation of eras of knowledge so the next leap can be made and yet remains the key back to that knowledge; or Pablo Neruda's words that can connect the personal to the universals of existential pain across vastly different cultures separated by language, geography, economics and history into a timeless, unboundaried space yet still be the gate back to the individual experience.

> I do not want to be the inheritor of so many misfortunes.
> I do not want to continue as a root and as a tomb,
> as a solitary tunnel, as a cellar full of corpses,
> stiff with cold, dying of pain.[8]

In my years of working with survivors of torture and extreme experiences I have always asked how the patients communicate their pain to themselves, in the privacy of their own world. In almost every case they have responded by saying they wrote poetry or stories, painted, drew, fixed things, made things. This question was inspired by the dedicated work on trauma treatment of several survivors of regimes in South America who had experienced periods of prolonged pain and torture as peoples and as states. These survivors were already or later became doctors, psychologists, therapists and social workers and advocated the use of metaphor in the treatment of torture. One of my cases was a man who was bereft of any colour in his life, incapable, he said, of any communication with himself about his truly horrific experiences. But he was pursued by nightmares so we used these as his communication, we worked with his nightmares as stories and significant progress was made in his recovery. Bruno Bettelheim, a survivor of the concentration camps who dedicated his life to working with autistic children, wrote a seminal work about the function of fairy tales in negotiating through the hazards and traumas of early life entitled *Tales of Enchantment and Meaning*.[9] To take a client back to a favourite child-time story can be the beginning of a revelation of the inner life of the person bypassing cognitive defences so that treatment interventions can be more appropriate.

To assist the medical and psychological practitioner in working with survivors of torture and extreme experiences by reducing the psychological and emotional pain which in turn often alleviates the physical, I would like to outline a few concepts to increase awareness which in turn can inform your practice. This does not mean changing how you do things, which may be incongruent with who you are, but they might help you to expand or push the boundaries a little further with patients with whom you feel you are making little progress. I can only hope to skim the surface of this complex but rewarding area in which to work, for these ideas have emerged out of practice, from the contributions of the patients themselves towards developing an understanding of the dynamics that can then provide the conditions of understanding which Hans-Georg Gadamer talks about. He was referring to Hermeneutics but it could just as well apply to any field of human interaction.

> Given the intermediate position in which hermeneutics operates, it follows that its work is not to develop a procedure of understanding but to clarify the conditions in which understanding takes place.[10]

MASLOW'S HIERARCHY OF NEEDS

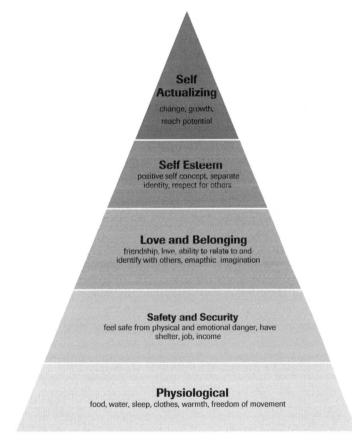

Figure 8.1 Maslow's hierarchy of needs

As systematic torture is based on a deprivation of Maslow's levels of needs, it is not surprising that to the survivor of torture the basic needs are essential – clothes, food, shelter. This may account for the high reports among practitioners that they are frustrated by patients being more interested in their housing or their day-to-day living events than the 'trauma'. It is these that were first removed, these things which constitute a solid base for any of us, and it is these that the patient is so desperate to put back in place and keep there. Torture destroys even the illusion of trust and creates intense uncertainty. If the definition of stress is uncertainty of outcome, then many survivors are among the most stressed people in society. If these basic needs are met, a survivor may still revert to insecurity around them as a paralanguage for the inability to move on to the safety and belonging needs (the relational) as these could be much more difficult to achieve. Firstly, they are in a foreign country, secondly, civil war has made them distrustful of others from their communities and/ or, thirdly, torture, which often attacks and perverts sexual functioning, has made them unworthy and in many cases dirty, shamed, different from others, cast out. In the case of survivors from Chile, the solidarity of the campaign in the UK, for example, provided many survivors with a community, a sense of belonging which contributed to relational recovery, the retention of identity and movement towards re-individuation. In many other communities, there is fragmentation rather than solidarity and this can embed the person in the lower levels of the Maslow hierarchy. In addition, survival has much to do with obsession with concrete detail which distracts the brain from the extreme anxiety of the existing pain or of more pain to come or from the sheer utter boredom and sensory deprivation, the waiting in nothingness, not knowing when you will ever be released. The 'permissible' actions, which are often just basic bodily functions, feed scraps to the brain of whatever it can find in this deprived place, until the thinking and the actions are almost rituals. This is to have a control over something because the greater terror cannot be controlled. How many tiles are in the cell, how many insects, what do they do, the intricate comparison of broken nails, marks on the skin …

> Always in the morning, I see the marks of the night's battle. Red lumps like chickenpox, all raging to be itched and scratched. I sit trying to prevent myself from scratching. The more I try to resist, the more difficult it becomes and the more demanding is my body for the exquisite pain of my nails tearing my own flesh. For some reason I do not understand, the feet and the backs of my fingers suffer the most from these insistent fleas. The pain of the bites on these tender areas can be excruciating. At times I exchange one pain for the other …[11]

I would like to note here that all of the above will be just as true for survivors of extreme experiences like childhood abuse. For a child whose fundamental safety and belonging needs have been betrayed, distorted and abused, they too, as they get older, will cling to the basic needs but these often become almost totally focused on the need for feeding (emotional and physical) which in turn is distorted into overfeeding, feeding through substances or self-harming behaviours or not feeding at all. To help the patient to ascend the hierarchy towards reintegration it is important to listen to and respect the issues of basic needs and rituals as a prelude to fuller engagement. The patient needs varied stimuli and not more of the same which the clinical room can be as can the attitude of the practitioner (*see* Metaphoric space on page 113). It can also be helpful to work with a locus of control (*see* Locus of control on page 110). Even if you think you are getting nowhere, the fact that the patient comes to you and you are there with a humanistic, relational attitude is reparative to the relational trust which has been so severely ruptured.

AUTHORITY DYNAMICS

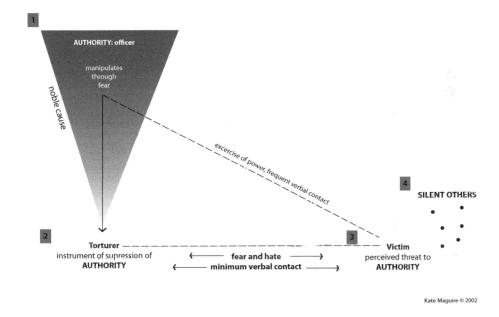

Kate Maguire © 2002

Figure 8.2 Torture relationship dynamic

Torture (and this includes childhood abuse and deprivation) is the inflicting of pain by one individual on another individual under the authority of the state, for a 'noble' cause or a belief system or a cultural/political system, or an entitlement embodied in an individual such as an officer, an elder, a religious figure or in an unchecked social or cultural norm like the right of parental authority over the child, the boss over the worker or the state over the individual. Therefore, effectively we can think of a torture/abuse dynamic of being principally a dynamic between four representational figures: Figure 1 the authority, Figure 2 the torturer, Figure 3 the victim and Figure 4 the silent others, those outside who do nothing to help. The activity of torture happens between Figure 2 and Figure 3. Figure 3 is terrified of Figure 2 and Figure 2 is terrified of Figure 1 because if he does not do his job well Figure 1 has the power to make him into a Figure 3. Figure 2 is encouraged by Figure 1 and Figure 2 aspires to and envies the authority of Figure 1. To Figure 3, Figure 2 is the demon, the psychopath beyond reason. In desperation, Figure 3 can project a benign image, a potential rescuer onto Figure 1, the authority, to which he or she can appeal for some sense, some reasonableness. Figure 1 remains aloof and powerful, appearing to keep his hands clean, a kind of Pontius Pilate archetype, while Figures 2 and 3 are effectively both victims. Milgram's experiments in the 1960s[12] illustrated this dynamic very well. Figure 4 remains constantly on the fringes like a question mark, the bad parent, the one who has turned his or her back. This Figure 4 is you and me. This dynamic is also one with parallels in terrorism, in the training and manipulation of terrorists where the noble cause is represented by the leaders and the foot soldiers carry out carnage among ordinary people (both are victims). In practice, it is important to see who you are for the patient in this authority dynamic and who the patient is for you and for him- or herself. Are you, as the practitioner, the torturer or the authority or the silent other? Is the patient afraid that he or she has become the torturer inflicting you with their terror, making you feel powerless like they were? This dynamic may help to understand the survivor's attitude to the practitioner, their transference and the clinician's counter-transference. Medical practitioners, because of their position and setting, can evoke transferences of either the torturer or the authority role depending on their attitude to the patient. Again understanding this dynamic can help the practitioner to see the value of a more humanistic, non-judgemental stance of positive regard and equality rather than anything than can be perceived to be pity, infantilising and patronising by the patient, evoking a range of responses from aggression to over-compliance and dependency.

DISAPPEARED

This term is well known in the field of torture and refers to the authorities 'disappearing' people by imprisoning them and/or brutally killing them but all the time denying their existence so no investigation can be carried out. It also refers to a form of torture in which the victim is hooded often for long periods of time and also during torture. This separates the individual from his or her world and denies the person their survival skill of anticipation. It also dehumanises the person in the eyes of the torturer. If they do not look into the victim's face they cannot be confronted by their own cruelty reflected there. When a person has been hooded for a long time, there is an adaptive response. The torturer cannot see the victim's face, their tears, their anger, their expression.

It can become a private, withdrawal place or the only means the individual can have of reacting against the torturer as the torturer cannot read the face. Even if a person has not been hooded during imprisonment, imprisonment itself is a form of being disappeared. The world goes on outside as normal and nobody and nothing is making this horror stop. People who have been tortured, abused and severely deprived have been disappeared by the rest of society, a society which is often justly perceived as having failed to prevent these terrible things from happening – the law, justice, other people, authorities, governments, international bodies. In practice, for some, pain can be a way to be visible, a scream in the dark, a way to be heard and subconsciously or unconsciously some can torture you with their scream and face you with their powerlessness so you know what it is like and will do something about it. For others physical pain is the acceptable face of an emotional pain which is often too shaming, too complex, too annihilating to be brought into the room. Many types of torture and abuse are both sexually invasive and designed to reach into the afterlife to deny that person any hope of redemption because they have been 'irreparably' morally corrupted. A victim often wants you to hear but does not want to turn into the abuser by forcing you to hear. For others, they withdraw (into the hood), they do not come out and scream until their coping behaviours become destructive and scream for them. In treating someone with this level of pain, it is important to be vigilant so that you do not hood or disappear them through a rushed appointment, a quick prescription, through not looking at them while they are speaking, having the minimum engagement, making the interval between appointments too long, not using their name, not listening, through being a Figure 4.

The following poem by an unnamed prisoner was smuggled out of La Libertad, a notorious prison in Uruguay which illustrates something of the complexities of being disappeared.

La Libertad

Today they took off my hood
How can I cry now?
Just at this very moment I so feel like crying
Where would I hide the tears now?
Now they have taken off my hood.

Some days this is what happens to me
I look for the word
and I can't find it
There must be one for sure
The Spanish language they say is so rich

Scrupulously I go over the length of my cell
There are fourteen tiles; but it's not there
I can't see it
I've got the concept clear
Of what I want to say
What I want to say to you

I look under the blanket
Just in case
The bastard's gone and hidden itself
but it's no use

I can't find the word
Because I would like to say
to say to you
to say to you
to say ...
I can't find the word.[13]

LOCUS OF CONTROL

A patient may appear to be dependent and powerless but that may not be the case in all areas of their life. A locus of control scale (*see* Figure 8.3) can be very revealing not only to the practitioner but also to the patient. It can, unlike some scales, be made by you the practitioner and presented in a user-friendly, respectful way as this scale is primarily not for the clinician but for the patient to give them a sense of their power, to see whether they are as powerless as they may feel. At one end of the scale is internal locus ('What I do makes a difference; I can get the environment to respond to me.') and at the other is external locus ('There is nothing I can do that will change things. It is not in my hands.'). It is not necessary to have analogue scales in between them. It is sufficient for the patient to put a mark or place a sticker along the line for each activity in their life. The most important information that the practitioner can give to the patient at the outset is that he or she must be a predominantly internal locused personality or they would not have survived torture and made it to this country (or, with regard to childhood abuse, survived abuse into adulthood). Circumstances, stress and pain all contribute to this locus becoming more externally focused but this scale often shows that the patient still has areas of his or her life in which the internal prevails. This visual representation of behaviours is enabling and provides a metaphor for the progress of sessions when the scale is revisited, when the patient has effected a change in their

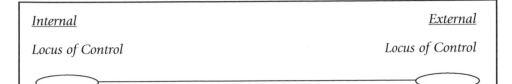

A belief that I can have an influence on the environment's responses to me, that I can influence the circumstances, that I can change myself and other things in my life

A belief that I can do nothing, it is in the hands of God, or authority, I have no power to alter the environment's response to me

Internal	External
Active	Passive
Empowerment	Disempowerment
Well being	Illness
Purpose	Depression
Socialisation	Isolation
Life	Death

1. The locus of control of any individual is not racially or culturally determined.
2. Experiences and environmental factors can greatly influence the position of the individual or the group along the scale.
3. It is not a fixed position but one that moves backwards and forwards during different stages of life.
4. It also moves in response to the impact of events (this is clinically very important when working with survivors of trauma).
5. We can have one position in relation to one thing and simultaneously take the opposite position in relation to another thing.
6. An individual can have one position and the group to which the individual belongs can have another creating tensions.
7. Sometimes what appears to be an external locus (there is nothing I can do) can in fact be internally locused if it is the most sensible option in the circumstances. For example, accepting there is nothing you can do about the traffic jam you are in and that you may as well enjoy the music rather than get frustrated and give yourself a heart attack.

Original concept Rotter[14]

Figure 8.3 Locus of control

life or behaviours or in someone else's life. The pain is often alleviated as the locus shifts more to the internal. I would just like to note here something on the issue of suicide and the locus of control. Suicide among survivors is not uncommon. Suicide is often seen as an act of despair, of powerlessness, coming from an external locus attitude – there is nothing I can do to change things, I am nothing in the world. Survivors of torture, whose whole experience of trauma has been about not having power, often speak about retaining one power that cannot be taken away from them, the power to choose whether to live or die and when. It is an act which, in this context, is motivated by an internal locus. Bettelheim, Primo Levi and others knew this well. Suicidal ideation or intent, therefore, is not straightforward when working with extreme experiences. In addition, standard clinical scales tend not to capture what I have called, for want of a better description, passive suicidal ideation, not uncommon among survivors of extreme experiences. This is when the patient has either cultural, religious or personal taboos against taking their own life or believes that if they actively take their own life then the torturers will have won. They may, therefore, subconsciously manipulate situations to die legitimately. Panic attacks may fall into this category as would reports of feeling faint and in danger of falling on a railway track or under a bus or feeling too ill to eat. It is often the pain of the shame and abandonment more than the physical pain that cannot be lived with and for many cannot be lived without as it is the testimony, the witness of what a human being is capable of. If one can recover from such abuse then it diminishes the severity of the act and of their pain.

METAPHORIC ENGAGEMENT

Practitioners are most successful with this client group if their attitude is person centred and humanistic. They can be analysts, psychodynamic therapists, pain specialists, doctors or dentists. It is not the approach that matters but the ability of the practitioner to be relational. The use of patient-led metaphors is simple and effective and manages to reduce rather than stimulate parallels of torture, intensification of sequelae and negative transference and counter-transference. It helps the patient not to have to put solely into words that which cannot be put into words and protects the practitioner from being vicariously abused by what is said. It also bypasses misunderstandings in the language. English is not often the first language of people who have been tortured. What does it involve? At the simplest level, it could be asking a client to draw or paint their pain or how they feel now. I had a client, a very well-educated man, who found it difficult to express anything about anything. I asked him if he could just draw something, anything, about how he was feeling at that moment. I gave him a pencil and paper. He drew a horizontal line. I asked him what it was. He said a desert. I asked him where he was. He said under the line. I asked him if he could breathe with all that sand. He said barely. Over time we used that line to see how he was feeling over the sessions and, over time, that picture developed until his head was above the sand and he could see birds. I asked him what kind of birds. He said maybe vultures or maybe there was an oasis near by and they were nice birds from there. He had not decided yet. Weeks later he drew an oasis. For some people favourite and hated colours are a metaphor. How are you today? A little yellow. I made a mistake once of thinking blue was a positive colour for a client because he just used it one sunny day and he had not associated this colour with any mood or feeling before. But it was later in the session when he revealed it was a colour he hated because it triggered flashbacks to a place in the prison where people were taken to be savaged by starving dogs and it was painted half blue and was splattered red with streaks of blood. Dreams, photos, objects, books, films, poetry, images, pictures and writings can all be used. They can be things the client has done or things they choose which they love or hate. The practitioner can use something like a chess set (or even a baskets of stones or shells) for family/relational dynamics – *which piece is you* (interestingly most patients choose the brown pawn). *Where would you like to put it on the board, which is your mother where would you like to put her, your father, brothers, sisters, gradually a person you really like, someone you hate,* etc. until a comprehensive picture is built up of a relational dynamic which would be very difficult to explain in words and any attempt would be exhausting even for a healthy person. Seeing the mapping on the chess board is helpful to both patient and practitioner and again this can be used in therapy to assess progress.

METAPHORIC SPACE

I mentioned earlier a link between the clinical room and the torture setting mainly in its lack of stimuli, its impersonal character. Even the practitioner can look and feel out of place. In the NHS, where I ran a trauma unit, we transformed the main clinical room into a metaphoric space. Patients would bring something to the room for the others who would visit there so that the objects and stories could be shared. In this space the therapist was the mediator not only between those in pain and those not, but also those in pain on different islands until there was a virtual community but held in reality by the room, the therapist, the objects and the stories. These patients never met but they were closer to each other than even to members of their own families. This reduced the isolation. The NHS room's transformation started with us buying an old table, a couple of comfortable chairs, an African art picture and mask and Indian cushions and a throw. Soon the room was full of ornaments. One of the patients took the old table away and mosaiced it, others hung their drawings, worry beads and dreamcatchers, some brought candles and flowers.

When the clinic was closed at weekends, the weekend staff used to take their breaks there because they loved it. This was the prison cell coming to life, where people could speak to each other, choose what stimulated their senses, make something beautiful from something barren, put new life into a place of pain, draw strength from each other.

I have asked my clients and patients if there was a pill to take the pain away would they take it. Those who have said yes have said as long as it does not take the memories away because someone has to bear witness. Those who have said no explain that such a pill would be like amputating something from them, some essential part of their reformed identity and they would no longer be able to be in solidarity with the people still being tortured in the world, they would be Figure 4s. In all my years of working in this field I have been humbled by the level of understanding and compassion survivors have for the human race, their striving to still find a way to connect, to go on. S once told me that he desperately wanted to take me to where he had been so I could really understand but would protect me with his life from ever going there. These people make considerable attempts to find their way back from those islands and we can give them the respect of meeting them half way, for their half of the journey has been agonising. When we truly encounter them, they, like Philoctetes, have significant knowledge to offer us in how we can help the others still stranded. It is an imperative of our humanity.

Again Remembrance

Slowly, slowly, the mist clears
From the shrouded glass
To reveal a splendour
Of naked reaching branches
Across a sunset flaming sky

And at the sun's bright setting
Their sad voices come
Through still and silent air
Their faces rise
Out of the blood light
And their hands like branches
All reach out to me

For this splendour was theirs
And this glory their eyes saw
And like them I do not want
To kill or die

So in the going down of this sun
I grieve
And in this evening remember
And with remembering resolve
Against all the odds – to love

To save this sunset for the ones to come
To sanctify this dying to the ones now gone

Philip Padfield
British hostage killed in Beirut 1986; written shortly before his kidnap[15]

REFERENCES

1 de Maupassant G. *The Horla and Other Stories.* Whitefish, MT: Kessinger Publishing Co; 2005.
2 Levi-Strauss C. *Structural Anthropology, Volume 2.* Layton M, trans. Harmonsdworth: Penguin; 1978. p. 54.
3 Scarry E. *The Body in Pain.* Oxford: Oxford University Press; 1987. p. 4.
4 Vinar M. A psychoanalytic look at torture. *British Journal of Psychotherapy.* 1989; 5(3): 359.
5 Sophocles. *Philoctetes.* 409 BCE. Trans. Francklin T. www.ancientgreece.com/s/People/Sophocles/
6 Words of a Holocaust survivor picked up on a radio programme in the 1990s.
7 Parry V. Why Pain can linger on the brain. In: Body and Soul section. *The Times.* 2008; 26 July. pp. 4–5.
8 Neruda P. Walking about. In: Neruda P. *Neruda: Selected Poems.* trans. Kerrigan A. Boston: Houghton Mifflin/Seymour Lawrence; 1990. p. 105.
9 Bettelheim B. *The Informed Heart.* London: Penguin Books Ltd; 1991. Preface, p. xii.
10 Gadamer H. In: Bruns G. *Hermeneutics Ancient and Modern.* New Haven: Yale University Press; 1992. p. 12.
11 Keenan B. *An Evil Cradling.* London: Vintage; 1993. p.64.
12 Milgram S. *Obedience to Authority.* New York: HarperCollins; 1974.
13 Anonymous. *La Libertad* [smuggled out of a Uruguayan prison of the same name].
14 Original concept: Rotter, J. *Social Learning and Clinical Psychology.* Englewood Cliffs, NJ: Prentice-Hall; 1954.
15 Padfield P. *Again Remembrance.* In: *Less than Complete.* Private publication. Maureen and Jan Bruns; 1992. Available from katemag@hotmail.co.uk

CHAPTER 9

Michelle

Andy Graydon

There is a Chinese story of a farmer who used an old horse to till his fields. One day the horse escaped into the hills and when the farmer's neighbours sympathised with the old man over his bad luck, the farmer replied, 'Bad luck? Good luck? Who knows?'. A week later the horse returned with a herd of horses from the hills and this time the neighbours congratulated him on his good luck. His reply was, 'Good luck? Bad luck? Who knows?'. Then when the farmer's son was attempting to tame one of the wild horses, he fell off its back and broke his leg. Everyone thought this was very bad luck. Not the farmer, whose only reaction was, 'Bad luck? Good luck? Who knows?'. Some days later the army marched into the village and conscripted every able-bodied youth they found there. When they saw the farmer's son with his broken leg they let him off. Now was that good luck? Bad luck? Who knows?

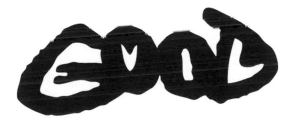

Like the image above, everything that seems on the surface to be an evil may well be a good in disguise. And everything that seems to be a good on the surface may really be an evil. So, perhaps, like the old Chinese farmer, we are wise to leave any form of judgement out of the equation. We just do not know. No one really knows what is good and what is bad – and it really does not matter what symbols we use: poverty, loneliness, loss, it is the concepts of good and bad that we attach them to that seems to make us suffer. Let me tell you about someone who seemed to live without these concepts.

Michelle died from cancer on 31 March 2007. She was a nurse at Tickhill Road Hospital. As a chaplain I used to see her for supervision every month, so we got to know each other fairly well. Over the years we talked quite a lot about everything. When she was nearing the end of her life she was taken into Weston Park, a cancer hospital in Sheffield. I decided to go to see her one Friday night when I felt that this particular visit could well be the last time we met together. Our last conversation was quite remarkable. She was sitting out of her bed in an armchair with her head laid on her arms, which were resting on one of those hospital tables. I asked if she was in pain, to which she answered, 'No, just knackered'. She found it hard to breathe so I said I would do most of the talking. I started our last conversation with the question: 'Do you still love your cancer?' To which she responded: 'Of course I do' Michelle came to love everything in the end. She was not one of those women who tried to 'fight' cancer, because she quickly came to realise that picking and choosing what you want to love is not really love at all, but self-interest. She knew that if she hated her cancer (as an evil) she could begin to reject anything or anyone who would not give her what she wants or threaten what she believes. No, she would love her cancer because it was part of who she was and therefore part of life. In doing so, she loved everything.

My second question was: 'Are you scared of dying?' She answered: 'No, not at all.' There was no negativity in her outlook. For Michelle, life was not about having jobs, money, possessions, etc., it was not even about being happy! All these things were her life's situations, which come and go, grow and die, chop and change. Michelle would even say: 'I do not have a life, I am life.' Whereas most people would see death as the opposite of life, Michelle could not accept that. For her the opposite of death was birth. She said she could observe the evidence of birth and death all around her: the seasons, the plants, animals, humans, planets, stars, solar systems, etc. So for Michelle, life has no opposite, life simply is – it is eternal, mystical and powerful. Death is part of the cycle of life, so why be scared of a cycle?

We would often talk about the analogy of a film. The projector throws light on to a screen and it produces images. There is only one light and many images. None of the images can exist without the light and indeed if the light disappeared all images would disappear with it. Everything that appears on the screen has no life force of its own. The characters on the screen along with the table and door, a mountain range or a cat have no substance of their own and depend on the light for their existence. Of course, we are not watching the film, we are the film, but nothing, none of us, not anything has any true being separate from the life force. The film expresses objects, characters, thoughts, ideas, dialogues – all of which come and go. Many are the times she would refer herself to being like a wave on the ocean. The wave has no identity separate from the ocean – it rises, sticks round for a while (in Michelle's case 38 years) and then returns to the ocean – nothing is truly lost. There is nothing tragic about that at all. It is part of the cycle. She would often remind me that every time I washed my face I would be destroying the lives of millions of microbes; and every year billions of our brain cells deteriorate and die – and nobody hardly notices or cares!

The third question was: 'Are there any regrets, anything you would have wanted to change at all Michelle?' She said: 'No, not a thing, everything is as it should be.' She certainly was a woman who accepted things as they are and not as she would like them to be. Not accepting the way things are was for her simply a recipe for unhappiness or disappointment. When I challenged her on this, I brought in her partner Cheryl, suggesting that surely she would have like to have spent a little more time with her. In no uncertain terms she retorted: 'You know that question is irrelevant Andy, and needless to say that you're missing the point. Accepting reality is all there is, and I am a lover of what is: I love sickness and health, coming and going, life and death. Reality is good, so death must be good. If you fight against reality – you lose – but only always [she would jest]! Cheryl will be all right.'

I kissed her goodbye and she died later that night.

WHAT I LEARNT FROM MICHELLE

Michelle taught me a lot about life and how to live it. Over the years I have reflected on how she has lived her life with cancer. Through knowing Michelle I have come to look at life in a completely new way and she has taught me quite a number of things. When I asked her, for instance, if she feared death, she would tell me: why fear a cycle – that is the way of nature and it is exactly what should happen. In one of our conversations we talked about how we have been conditioned in our mind-dominated Western world to overstress the apparent separateness of things in life. Of course, this concept is very practical for everyday living, but it needs to be balanced by an awareness of an underlying reality which holds everything together. After all we live in a universe (uni – meaning one, of course). There is an oneness that gives life to everything that is. This is true of who we are. It is certainly clear that we are not our body, and we are not our mind, we are not our emotions and we are certainly not who we say we are. Who we are goes beyond any mind concepts we have about who we are. None of these have any substance of their own. It is the one abiding presence; this intelligent oneness that keeps blood pumping around my body, that makes my finger nails and hair grow, is the same life force that makes the trees grow, keeps the sun burning and the planets spinning round it.

Another area that Michelle helped me to focus on was the apparent distinction we make between the past and the future. Again, this has very practical uses in everyday life, but in reality past and future have no real substance of their own. Eckhart Tolle once said:

> Imagine the earth devoid of human life, inhabited only by plants and animals. Would it still have a past and a future? Could we still speak of time in any meaningful way? The question What time is it? Or what's today's date? – if there was anyone to ask it – would be quite meaningless. The oak tree or eagle would be bemused by such a question. 'What time?' they would ask. 'Well, of course, it's now. The time is now. What else is there?'[1]

Michelle was able to express this kind of living in practically all her relationships. Honesty and empathy were the hallmarks of Michelle's life. She knew how to build bridges with people and she would often remind me that if we are not building bridges, then we are, by default, building walls!

BRIDGE BUILDING AND SINCERITY

Let's take a look at this bridge building in further detail. If the bridge is to be solid and stable it is essential that the self end of the bridge is the genuine article. This involves honesty, or perhaps a better word sincerity. The word sincere is derived from the Latin *sine* (without) and the Greek *cera* (wax), which refers to the ancient custom of covering up broken marble statues with wax and selling them as intact – hence *sine cera* – sincere, without pretence. There are two kinds of sincerity: outer (or intellectual) and inner (or emotional). Outer sincerity is about intellectual integrity: doing what is right, following the rules and moral codes, etc. Divergence from this is insincerity: we hate and despise liars and easily and intuitively recognise one. Lying in this context consists of expressing something that you do not in fact truly think, pretending to believe something that you in fact do not accept. We could call this negative insincerity. But, of course, there is more to honesty than refraining from lying. So, when we fail to express what we do believe or think to someone when it would be to their advantage to know, it could be seen as being guilty of positive insincerity.

Now, inner (emotional) sincerity is both more important and more difficult to live out. Again, it is best defined by its obverse insincerity, which can be negative or positive. We are guilty of negative insincerity if we express a feeling, such as love, when in fact we do not truly feel it. Positive emotional insincerity is when we fail to express what we truly feel to a person when it might make a real difference to them. True inner sincerity is much more difficult to achieve than we imagine. In contrast to outer (intellectual) insincerity, which is sometimes excused, for example, when trying to protect someone or you tell a lie because of fear for self, it would never be commended; yet emotional insincerity is often regarded as a duty! The concealment of feelings or pretence of having emotions that are not felt is even encouraged as a social virtue!

We are on dangerous ground here. When we pretend with our feelings we are at the risk of losing the capacity to distinguish between truth and falsehood and so deceive ourselves about what we believe. If we cheat others about our feelings we may soon become unable to know what we really feel. For instance if we tell ourselves that we may love someone what we in fact do not, we may actually end up believing that we love them, but unconsciously hating them. Such loss of emotional integrity not only weakens existing relationships, but also prevents any true relationships from blossoming.

To disguise how we feel will, in any case, rarely succeed. And it will rarely convince other people. In an office of secretaries at Medical Records, when a new girl arrived one of the previously existing team took a dislike to her and would constantly make negative comments about her when she was not there, but yet be seemingly pleasant when she was there. One day she spoke up and said to the woman in question: 'Why do you hate me so much, what have I done?' The woman who had made the backbiting comments failed to recognise that her pretence did not fool the new girl. No matter how much you pretend to love someone, if in fact you have no real love for that person, it will usually show!

I once, in the local hospice, heard a spouse saying to her dying partner: 'Oh, you will be up playing football tomorrow! You are looking a lot better today.' In fact, both no doubt were 'hiding' their true feelings, for fear they may 'hurt' each other. The after-effects of not being truly open and honest run deeply in the heart of the remaining spouse with a pain that rarely heals. They carry with them a sorrowful form of regret that usually clings to them to the grave.

Michelle lived a life of inner and outer sincerity and was open and honest in everything and with everyone. She was a constant challenge to those around her who may have thought otherwise in their own relationships. In this way Michelle was able to teach us all so much, even from her own deathbed!

It was through my relationship with Michelle that the idea of offering all members of staff in the trust where I work a chance to take part in a residential experience that came to be called 'A Self-Awareness Course'. It is aimed at enabling members of staff to cope more effectively with the stresses of modern living and the tensions which arise in the work and home environment. The three-day timetable, while allowing plenty of time for relaxation, is made up largely of reflective exercises and discussions aimed a promoting a deeper sense of personal awareness and a capacity for warm, open and accepting relationships. In an environment where a warm and accepting atmosphere is obvious among the staff, it will be easier to promote a more holistic approach to physical and emotional healing of patients. The course has been running for 10 years and over 250 members of staff have benefited from it.

I remind the participants that the self-awareness course is likewise, time for themselves – time to enjoy themselves. Not just enjoying doing things or other people's company, but really enjoying who they really are. For some who do not think too highly of themselves, this often proves a problem. One of the most significant parts of the course is a session we do on mask-wearing. We show them a 15-minute film strip (cartoon like) called 'In-the-Bin', about people who all wear masks and in particular about one man – Arthur Stanley Grimble. He will find a mask to fit every situation – a mask for best, for a snarl, for sympathy, for kindness, for firmness, etc. A dustman, a man without a mask who carries his own dustbin, constantly follows him. Eventually he confronts Arthur and empties his cupboard of all the masks he possesses and even takes off the mask he is wearing, and they all go in the bin – every last one! The film strip ends up with poor Arthur making a new order for more masks; life without a mask would be more frightening than living with one! This provokes excellent discussion and opens up some very revealing stories of why and when people wear masks themselves. Throughout the course we do an amazing amount of uncovering of masks ourselves. The exercises open up the whole process of sincere communication, which seems essential to living life to the full. I am grateful to Michelle for teaching me so much. She was one of the first to attend a self-awareness course and I have learned so much from her ever since.

It was only two years after Michelle died that her partner Cheryl, was herself diagnosed with breast cancer, as was Michelle six years previously. Cheryl is doing fine at the moment and she has recently been remarried in a civil service. Michelle would have deeply approved.

REFERENCE

1 Tolle E. *The Power of Now*. Novato, CA: New World Library; 1999. Hodder Mobius; 2005 edition. pp. 27–8.

CHAPTER 10

Recovery from alcoholism and other addictions: a model for managing spiritual pain

Paul D Martin and Paul Bibby

(This chapter is largely based on a paper published by one of the authors.[1])

Reflection on what it means to be a healthcare professional and indeed a patient, the dynamic giving and receiving between both parties and the aims of care rather than cure by the authors and others has led to recognition of some of the common features between people who are living with long-term benign pain and those recovering from alcoholism. This chapter is an investigation of possible parallels not only of the shared features of spiritual suffering but also of the possibility of shared options for therapy and healing. The authors explore the concepts of powerlessness, acceptance, transition and its subsequent growth and healing with subsequent relief of spiritual pain through acceptance, a sense of powerlessness, forgiveness, making amends, development of a relationship with a 'power greater than ourselves', in areas of their diseases, health, relationships and human activity.

INTRODUCTION

> Alcoholics Anonymous is a fellowship of men and women who share their experience strength and hope with each other that they may solve their common problem and help others recover from alcoholism.

These words are part of the preamble read out at over 100 000 regular Alcoholics Anonymous (AA) group meetings held in over 150 countries worldwide with an excess of 2 million active participants.[2-4]

While various models of alcoholism have been described, the disease model[5] is now widely accepted[6-8] and has been extensively researched with the conclusion that participation in the fellowship of AA is associated with improvement in physical, psychological, emotional, spiritual and social well-being and is as good as if not more successful than other therapies.[9,10]

The recognition that alcoholism and other addictions have their expression in these physical, psychological, emotional, spiritual and social consequences and that the principles of recovery espoused by AA addresses each of these invites the notion that such an approach may be therapeutic in other diseases.

THE HISTORY AND DEVELOPMENT OF ALCOHOLICS ANONYMOUS

In April 1935 Bill Wilson, a chronic drunk and businessman from New York was visiting Akron Ohio for the purpose of securing contracts. In the evening he stood outside the bar of his hotel with an overwhelming craving to drink, but instead he telephoned several religious organisations seeking to find another chronic drunk with whom he could speak. He was introduced to a local surgeon, Bob Smith, similarly afflicted. At this meeting there occurred identification with each other and a friendship established. They found that by sharing their experiences, feelings and thoughts with each other they could remain sober. Subsequently they sought out other drunks who could not achieve the sobriety they desperately sought. Many did not take the opportunity to share and the attrition rate was high. But many did and thus the Fellowship of Alcoholics Anonymous came into being.

Four years later this expanding group sought to analyse how they were achieving the sobriety and health that had hitherto eluded them. This they recorded in a book and the first edition of *The Big Book* was published.[3] Now in its fourth edition (the third edition having sold in excess of 12 million copies), it comprises a collection of personal stories including those of Bill Wilson and Bob Smith. In addition it sets out the principles common to those who found sobriety this way – 'The Twelve Steps'.

Alcoholics who come to the fellowship of AA learn to:

➤ make a decision on a daily basis not to drink alcohol
➤ attend AA meetings frequently and regularly
➤ be sponsored by more experienced, longer sober individuals (who themselves are sponsored) and proceed to sponsor others
➤ 'work' the Twelve Steps.

ANALYSIS OF RECOVERY PRINCIPLES

The daily decision to abstain from alcohol represents a defined manageable period – tomorrow is another day and the decision today does not apply tomorrow. Such a process has been described for other circumstances and can be expressed as 'keeping it in the moment'. Similarly its therapeutic place is being described in other illnesses and diseases as well as life activities as 'mindfulness'.[11,12]

Frequent and regular attendance at AA meetings provides social activity, mutual support from and to persons with similar experiences as well as reinforcement of personal commitment through encouragement and example both for the attendee and also from the attendee to others. This latter principle is described as 'service' and can be alternatively described as altruism.

Sponsorship acts similarly but is a closer, more involved relationship with another recovering alcoholic often with daily contact and communication and has a mentoring and guidance aspect. It is important that sponsors are themselves sponsored and sponsees also become sponsors.

THE TWELVE STEPS

Step 1

> We admitted that we were powerless over alcohol – that our lives had become unmanageable.

This addresses what has been described as a faulty belief system concerning the power of self and control. In psychological terms it is a recognition of ego boundaries[13] and a breaking of the protective mechanism of denial. Step 1 also acknowledges negative and destructive consequences as evidence of that loss of control and powerlessness.

Step 2

> We came to believe that a power greater than ourselves could restore us to Sanity.

This step builds on the first in suggesting that having accepted that alcohol was more powerful than the person, there could be an even greater power, greater than alcohol and that this could be accessed. This step also represents an introduction to a spiritual experience of recovery.[13-15] A significant element of this aspect of recovery is related to the admission that restoration of 'sanity' is desirable, inferring that the individual may have an altered perception of reality.

Step 3

> We made a decision to turn our will and lives over to the care of God as we understand Him.

This is an example of cognitive restructuring with further deflation of ego and self-will and the establishment and commitment to a spiritual experience and relationship, accepting the challenge of trust and a letting go of control.[13]

Step 4

We made a searching and fearless moral inventory of ourselves.

This is an example of reflection of who the person is and what determines that sense of personhood. It requires a commitment to rigorous honesty and again dissembles the ego-defending mechanism of rationalising.[15]

Step 5

We admitted to God, to ourselves, and to another human being the exact nature of our wrongs.

This reinforces the spiritual experience of relationships with others and a higher power and the fundamental need and reward of communications with others and the cosmos – a placement of self in the community, in society and in a greater perspective.

Step 6

We were entirely ready to have God remove all these defects of character.

This builds on that sense of perspective and invites transformation and change and a shift from wilfulness to willingness.[13–15]

Step 7

We humbly asked Him to remove our shortcomings.

This is an active step in the spirit of faith and a development of humility.[13–15]

Step 8

We made a list of all persons we had harmed, and became willing to make amends to them.

This is the first tangible move towards relocating self and responsibility as an individual and participant in community, society and real life. The concept of giving and receiving forgiveness introduced in Steps 5, 6 and 7 becomes more explicit and tangible.

Step 9

> We made direct amends to such people whenever possible, except where to do so would injure them or others.

This moves to repair and restore damage and lays the foundation for renewal and further growth from past actions as well from new and future experiences. The sense of asking for and offering forgiveness becomes a reality.

Step 10

> We continued to take a personal inventory and when we were wrong promptly admitted it.

This is a continuation of Step 4 and a means of maintaining a sense of self, appreciation of its fragility and the value of timely attention to movements away from contentment and health.

Step 11

> We sought through prayer and meditation to improve our conscious contact with God as we understand Him, praying only for knowledge of His will for us and the power to carry that out.

This serves as active spiritual expression and perspective of self.[14-16]

Step 12

> Having had a Spiritual Awakening as a result of working these steps, we tried to carry this message to alcoholics and to practice these principles in all our affairs.

This confirms the recognition of the individual as a spiritual being with relationships outside self. In addition it introduces the concept of service to others and confirms the notion that the problem is the person not the alcohol and as such the solution is applicable to other aspects of a person's life, actions, feelings, thoughts and relationships.[15,16]

The daily decision to abstain from alcohol, the admission of powerlessness, acceptance, ego deflation , reflection, identification of personhood, spiritual awakening, development of a relationship with others and a higher power and place of self in those relationships with subsequent transformation through forgiveness, ownership, responsibility, service and altruism all serve to address the alcoholics' suffering of the physical, psychological, emotional, spiritual and social sources of their disease and thereby return to health and the prospect of remission from that disease.

RECOVERY AND HOLISTIC HEALING

Healing can be compared to pain or love, in the sense that most people know what it means but it remains difficult to describe, and as such is subjective and intimate, at the same time as being a universal experience. Palliative medicine literature has sought to describe healing at life's end.[17] Mount and Kearney have stated that, 'it is possible to die healed'. They go further to suggest that while healing may be facilitated by a caregivers intentions it is 'dependant on an innate potential'. That is to say healing comes from within, the issue is the person not just the disease – a realisation essential to Twelve Step recovery. We contend that spiritual pain comes from the person, not necessarily the disease or physical pathology.

Descriptors of healing such as relational and connectedness are emerging in the health literature and are also supported in thoughts around the new physics[18] as well as historically and through arts and the humanities.[19] Such language and concepts are identifiable to and resonates with those recovering from alcoholism and utilising the programme of AA. In a paper on the rhetoric of transformation in the healing of alcoholism, Swora has suggested that, 'healing is not a cure, but a new way of attending to the world and engaging with others, including God, or a Power greater than Ourselves'.[20]

HEALING FROM ALCOHOLISM AND OTHER DISEASES

The success of AA for the healing from alcoholism is well documented.[10,11] Vaillant in particular has summarised the studies and mechanisms of the efficacy of AA and reports that recovering alcoholics 'lived longer, had better mental health, better marriages, were more responsible parents and were more successful employees'.[21]

Moreover the principles have been adopted for other addictions with the establishment of groups such as Narcotics Anonymous, Gamblers Anonymous, Sex and Love Addicts Anonymous. There are even groups for specific disease states including HIV Anonymous and Hepatitis C Anonymous. There are also groups for those related or close to the primary sufferers (Al-Anon for partners and spouses of alcoholics, Al-Ateen for children of alcoholics and Families Anonymous for relatives of drug addicts) all of which adopt AA principles for the return to and maintenance of health and lives affected by relationships with the primary patients.

There exists a renewed and increasing recognition and attention to health issues as being more than pathophysiological abnormalities with dysfunction of biological systems and any therapies directed solely at those abnormal pathologies.[18,22–24]

Keefe has reported the benefits of spiritual activity in living with rheumatoid arthritis.[25] Carson describes the relationship between forgiveness and chronic low back pain[26] and Hutchinson, in a study of transitions in patients with end-stage renal disease, has offered the notion of a need of a safe place to suffer during transitions (c.f. the community of the fellowship of AA) and such a place can result in healing.[27] Greer in his paper 'Healing the mind/body split: bringing the patient back into oncology'[23] calls for the biomedical model to be enlarged to include psychosocial factors and stresses that, 'medical care requires treatment not only of the disease but of the patient who suffers from the disease' and illustrates this with case studies in cancer sufferers. Reporting on survivors from prostate cancer Bowie identifies spiritual experience and activity as improving quality of life.[28]

'RECOVERY' FROM SPIRITUAL PAIN

The International Association for the Study of Pain defines pain as: 'A sensory and emotional experience associated with actual or potential tissue damage or described in terms of such damage.'

Chronic pain, like other long-term health problems, is often associated with psycho-social co-morbidities.[29] These are not dissimilar to what are described within AA literature as the 'soul-sickness' of alcoholism. As described by Bibby many others apart from addicts display 'an existential conflict that seems insatiable'.[30]

The disease of living with the pain that life is (be that associated with a physical, e.g. lower back pain, or meta-physical, e.g. memory of abuse, manifestation) can be such that the person becomes a slave to the pain which ostensibly becomes their 'Higher Power'. The application of the principles of the Twelve Steps into scenarios such as chronic pain and palliative care is to assist the sufferer in addressing their pain specifically from the spiritual perspective. Interestingly, mindfulness – a form of acceptance-based meditation, which is based on Buddhist meditation – is becoming increasingly practised within both pain management services as a form of cognitive behavioural therapy and by recovering addicts seeking to improve their relationship with a higher power.

Acceptance has been shown to be related to physical healing and recovery in survivors of landmine explosions resulting in traumatic amputation.[31] A reframing process occurs resulting in psychological healing when forgiveness is practiced.[32-34] Finally, altruism is associated with well-being, happiness, health and longevity.[35,36]

SUMMARY

The disease of alcoholism can be halted by involvement with and participation in the fellowship of AA. The programme of recovery offered by AA addresses the physical, psychological, emotional, spiritual and social constituents of the disease in a holistic sense. It is suggested that it may be possible to adapt the program to other diseases such that ill people may similarly benefit from the following.

1. Making a daily decision of acceptance of their disease.
2. Communicating with others with similar afflictions.
3. Seeking guidance from and providing guidance to others suffering.
4. Activating innate healing by adopting the AA approach, for example, paraphrasing the first step:

> We admitted we were powerless over our pain, terminal illness, bipolar disorder, infertility, etc. …

A healing may be experienced through transformation from powerlessness to a sense of acceptance, identification of self, application of rigorous honesty, humility, ownership and responsibility. The practice of forgiveness, development of a sense of spirituality, defining relationship to others and to the universe and acting in service in the spirit of altruism all offer the prospect of healing and contentment with life's rigours including illness and even death.

REFERENCES

1 Martin PD. Healing from alcoholism and other addictions – a model for holistic health care. *British Journal of Holistic Healthcare*. 2006; **3**(4): 19–24.
2 Bewley AR. Addiction and meta-recovery: wellness beyond the limits of Alcoholics Anonymous. *Alcoholism Treatment Quarterly*. 1993; **10**(1–2): 1–22.
3 Alcoholics Anonymous. *Alcoholics Anonymous*. 4th ed. New York: Alcoholics Anonymous World Services Inc.; 2001.
4 www.alcoholics-anonymous.org/en_media_resources.cfm?PageID=75
5 Jellinek EM. *The Disease Concept of Alcoholism*. New York: Hillhouse Press; 1960.
6 Kurtz E. Alcoholics Anonymous and the disease concept of alcoholism. *Alcoholism Treatment Quarterly*. 2002; **20**(3–4): 5–40.
7 American Psychiatric Association. *Diagnostic and Statistical Manual of Mental Disorders*. 4th ed. (DSM-IV). Washington, DC: American Psychiatric Association; 1994.
8 World Health Organization. *International Classification of Disease Tenth Revision, Clinical Modification (ICD-10-CM)*. Geneva: World Health Organization; 2003.
9 Vaillant GE. Alcoholics Anonymous: cult or cure? *Australia and New Zealand Journal of Psychiatry*. 2005; **39**: 431–6.
10 McIntire D. How well does AA work? An analysis of published AA surveys (1968–1996) and related analyses/comments. *Alcoholism Treatment Quarterly*. 2000; **18**(4):1–18;
11 Hutchinson TA. Coming home to mindfulness in medicine. *Canadian Medical Association Journal*. 2005; **173**(4): 391–3.
12 Schmidt S. Mindfulness and healing intention: concepts practice and research evaluation. *Journal of Alternative and Complementary Medicine*. 2004; **10**(1): S7–14.

13 Steigerwald F, Stone D. Cognitive restructuring and the 12-Step Program of Alcoholics Anonymous. *Journal of Substance Abuse Treatment.* 1999; **16**(4): 321–7.

14 Lile B. Twelve Step programs: an update. *Addiction Disorders and their Treatment.* 2003; 2: 19–24.

15 Naifeh S. Archetypal foundations of addiction and recovery. *Journal of Analytical Psychology.* 1995; **40**: 133–59.

16 Carroll S. Spirituality and purpose in life in alcoholism recovery. *Journal of Studies on Alcohol.* 1993; **54**(3): 297–301.

17 Mount B, Kearney M. Healing and palliative care: charting our way forward. *Palliative Medicine.* 2003; **17**: 657–8.

18 Berger LS. Psychotherapy, biological psychiatry and the nature of matter: a view from physics. *American Journal of Psychotherapy.* 2001; **55**(2): 185–201.

19 Evans HM, Greaves D. Medial humanities among the healing arts. *Medical Humanities.* 2002; **28**(2): 57–60.

20 Swora MG. The Rhetoric of transformation in the healing of alcoholism: the twelve steps of Alcoholics Anonymous. *Mental Health, Religion and Culture.* 2004; **7**(3): 187–209.

21 Vaillant GE. A 60 year follow up of male alcoholism. *Addiction.* 2003; **98**: 1043–51.

22 Bracken P, Thomas P. Time to move beyond the mind body split. *British Medical Journal.* 2002; **325**: 1433–4.

23 Greer S. Healing the mind/body split: bringing the patient back into oncology. *Integrative Cancer Therapies.* 2003; **2**(1): 5–12.

24 Galanter M. Spiritual recovery movements and contemporary medical care. *Psychiatry.* 1997; **60**(3): 211–23.

25 Keefe FJ, Affleck G, Lefebre J, *et al.* Living with rheumatoid arthritis: the role of daily spirituality and daily religious and spiritual coping. *The Journal of Pain.* 2001; **2**(2):101–10.

26 Carson JW, Keefe FJ, Fras AM, *et al.* Forgiveness and chronic low back pain: a preliminary study examining the relationship of forgiveness to pain, anger and psychological distress. *The Journal of Pain.* 2005; **6**(2): 84–91.

27 Hutchinson TA. Transitions in the lives of patients with end stage renal failure: a cause for suffering and an opportunity for healing. *Palliative Medicine.* 2005; **19**: 270–7.

28 Rowie JV, Sydnor KD, Granot M, *et al.* Spirituality and coping among survivors of prostate cancer. *Journal of Psychosocial Oncology.* 2004; **22**(2): 41–56.

29 Schofield P. Effects of chronic pain. In: Schofield P (ed). *Beyond Pain.* London: Whurr; 2005.

30 Bibby P. Alcoholism and addiction: the management of spiritual pain in the clinical environment. In: Schofield P (ed). *Beyond Pain.* London: Whurr; 2005.

31 Ferguson AD. Psychological factors after traumatic amputation in landmine survivors: the bridge between physical healing and full recovery. *Disability and Rehabilitation.* 2004; **26**(14–15): 931–8.

32 Hope D. The healing paradox of forgiveness. *Psychotherapy.* 1987; **24**(2): 240–4.

33 Worthington EL, Jr, Witvliet C van O, Lerner A, *et al.* Forgiveness in health research and medical practice. *Explore – The Journal of Science and Healing.* 2005; **1**(3): 169–76.

34 Lawler KA, Younger JW, Piferi RL, *et al.* The unique effects of forgiveness on health: an exploration of pathways. *Journal of Behavioural Medicine.* 2005; **28**(2):157–67.

35 Post SG. Altruism, happiness and health: it's good to be good. *International Journal of Behavioural Medicine.* 2005; **12**(2): 66–77.

36 Scwartz CE. Altruistic social interest behaviours are associated with better mental health. *Psychosomatic Medicine.* 2003; **65**(5): 778–85.

CHAPTER 11

Learning to accept suffering

Peter Wemyss-Gorman

Suffering seems to be an inevitable component of the human condition. It is universal, has always existed and presumably always will. Understanding it has been a major preoccupation of all philosophies and religions. Although the answers to questions such as 'Why is there suffering?' or 'Is suffering compatible with belief in a loving God?' may be beyond our understanding, one thing is plain to see: we can in no way escape the relentless evidence that it is inevitable. We simply have to accept this, however reluctant we may be. But from shamans and witch doctors to the physicians of ancient Greece and mediaeval Arabia, through the Enlightenment and the rise of scientific medicine down to the present day and the emergence of pain relief as a specialty, all the activities of the healing professions are predicated on the principle that pain and suffering are *un*acceptable.

(Michael Bavidge has written elsewhere in this book about the difference between pain and suffering – *see* Chapter 2 on page 31. There are obviously other causes of suffering than pain and although this chapter is mainly focused on pain, much of it can be extrapolated to other forms of suffering.)

Pain is of course not all inevitable. Most acute pain, pain due to cancer and some chronic non-malignant pain can usually be relieved by simple and straightforward measures such as analgesics. Well-established chronic pain can be much more difficult and unrewarding to treat, but more sophisticated physical and pharmacological interventions do quite frequently work, and provide at least temporary respite and sometimes long-lasting relief. But sadly all too often they do not. Surely the huge amount of research that has been going on all round the world for the last 30 years and more and the enormous advances in understanding of the workings of the nervous system will one day bear fruit in terms of more effective treatment? Looking at the number of useful spin-offs to date would hardly encourage unqualified optimism but it would surely be wrong to admit defeat and abandon the search.

The fact that pain is sometimes preventable and can sometimes be relieved makes acceptance of it and failure to relieve it all the more difficult. I would guess that for many doctors, especially those engaged in pain medicine, learning to accept their limitations is one of the most challenging aspects of growing into the job. In my early days in pain management, when my results never seemed to come up to expectations I attributed it to incompetence and got pretty despondent. Then I gradually began to realise that my expectations, and those I had encouraged in my patients, were very often unrealistic.

However difficult it may be, it is still necessary to accept the inevitability of suffering and will remain so for the foreseeable future. But although acceptance must include acknowledging the inevitable it does not necessarily imply passivity, as resignation does. Nor is it the same as endurance, which implies toughness, bravery and not giving way; or stoicism, which implies acceptance of pain or hardship without display of feelings or complaint. These may be admirable and valuable qualities but – fortunately for the majority of us – they are not indispensable in our present context. As we shall see, acceptance can be something not only positive and helpful, but also accessible even to the least stoical of us.

ACCEPTANCE AND RELIGION

The prayer for serenity goes some way to expressing this sense of acceptance:

> God, give us grace to accept with serenity the things that cannot be changed, courage to change the things that should be changed, and the wisdom to distinguish the one from the other.

People everywhere have always looked to religion to help them to accept their suffering. Michael Hare Duke discusses how much religions help us to understand the mysteries of suffering in another chapter (*see* Chapter 3 on page 41), but I am concerned here with the place of religion in helping us to accept suffering. There are two contrasting strands. The first is to be found in the Abrahamic, monotheistic religions that require belief in an omnipotent God who knows what is best for us, and has a loving purpose for us, however contrary to appearances this may be. This is perhaps seen in its purest form in Islam, which is entirely predicated on acceptance of and obedience to the will of Allah. However unacceptable this idea may seem to non-religious people, countless millions throughout the ages, including many of those who have experienced life's cruellest blows, have found solace and comfort in it, and the will to go on in the darkness.

The other strand, found in the oriental religions of Hinduism and especially Buddhism, does not require belief in an omnipotent deity, and is perhaps more attractive to the modern secular mind. It is also the basis for one approach to the practical management of intractable pain. Buddhism is indeed *all* about suffering: the Buddha said, 'all I teach is suffering and the deliverance from suffering'. The dense complexities of Buddhist teaching are beyond the scope of this chapter (and indeed the comprehension of its author) and the reader is directed to the Further reading section (*see* page 139) for guidance in these. Its basic message is, however, relatively simple and summed up in The First Noble Truth: *there is suffering*. The Second Noble Truth is concerned with the cause of suffering, and states that suffering arises from attachment and aversion: our need for things to be or not to be in a certain way, and especially our aversion to the way things are. It involves resistance, struggle and trying to shut off experience. Suffering is what happens when we struggle with whatever our life experience is rather than accepting it with a wise and compassionate response. Suffering can only be successfully dealt with (the Third Noble Truth) by letting go of attachment and aversion to what is, and letting go of our defensive and protective strategies, the armour we put on to shield ourselves from reality. This is of course totally counterintuitive, and seems opposed to evolution. We are hard-wired to protect ourselves, to survive.

The Buddha prescribed a Noble Eightfold Path to achieving this aim, in which the most important element, in the present context, is mental discipline. This includes mindfulness and meditation as the means for investigating our experience and reality and for being present with what is. Mindfulness has been defined as awareness of one's thoughts, actions or motivations and involves bringing one's awareness back (i.e. from the past or the future) into the present moment by concentrating on sensate experience, initially that of breathing, and eventually even the sensation of pain. It aims to exclude, or rather recognise and put on one side, the chatter of thoughts, so often pessimistic and catastrophic, which accompany the experience of suffering and the narratives we invent in a futile and counterproductive attempt to 'protect' ourselves. Although it is usually thought of as something which can only be achieved in a meditative state, it is also a mode of thought which can be cultivated and used at any time.

TEACHING ACCEPTANCE IN CHRONIC PAIN MANAGEMENT

For the past few decades, pain management programmes (designed to help people to live productive and enjoyable lives despite pain that cannot be relieved, and usually run by teams of psychologists, physiotherapists, occupational therapists and specialist nurses) have become a mainstay of pain services. Although their original *raison d'être* lay in the limitations of 'physical' therapies this has more and more been superseded by recognition of the fact that pain affects a human being, body mind and spirit, as a whole and needs 'holistic' treatment. Awareness and correction of maladaptive thoughts and behaviour is an important component of the pain management approach. In recent years there has been an increasing emphasis on helping patients to accept their pain and acknowledge the futility of pursuing the search of cure for it.

Like Buddhism, acceptance and commitment therapy (ACT) is based on the idea that suffering comes less from the experience of pain, whether physical or emotional, than from our attempted avoidance of that pain. Its goal is to help people to focus less on trying to escape or avoid pain (because this is impossible) and more on regaining the capacity to live a meaningful life in spite of it. Acceptance on this view does not imply simply resigning oneself to suffering. Rather it involves acknowledging the reality that it may be necessary to face some pain if it is the price one has to pay for pursuing worthwhile and practical goals and activities. It involves acknowledging that thoughts and feelings may unnecessarily hold one back in this pursuit. Mindfulness as outlined above is a widely used means of achieving this aim.

Acceptance restores the freedom to choose priorities to those who feel that their pain has robbed them of choice. It is of course not incompatible with other pain management and control strategies. It does not exclude 'medical' interventions where these have been found to be at least partially useful, provided that the single-minded, desperate but futile search for a medical cure is abandoned. Although I said earlier that it is accessible to the least stoical, I did not mean to imply that it is always easy. Not only does it require changing a mindset that has accreted over years, but also resistance to the daily temptation to return to old ways of thought and reaction to pain. Nevertheless acceptance is the essential starting point for all the processes of rebuilding lives that pain management offers.

ACCEPTANCE OF OTHER PEOPLE'S SUFFERING

So much for patients accepting their own pain. But what about us in the healing professions? What about *our* acceptance of *other people's* pain? Our whole ethos is built around our duty to relieve suffering so does acceptance of another's pain relieve us of that duty? Acceptance can never mean simply giving up: 'I've accepted his pain and told him he must accept it so that's all right then – next patient please.' On the other hand, accepting another's suffering may guard us from the desperation to do *something* that may lead us to excessive or inappropriate treatment. The temptation to try just one more treatment which might just work, or repeat an intervention one might just possibly have done incorrectly the first time, can be reinforced both by the patient's distress and by the experience that once in a while this was the right thing to do, even when we know the chances of success are tiny and all we are doing is postponing acceptance. A recent study of high-dose opioid prescribing in patients with chronic pain showed that they were most likely to be used in patients with multiple pain and psychological problems, and had the highest risk of a poor outcome. It was suggested that that these are the most distressed patients, with the greatest desperation for relief, and doctors meet their demands by prescribing opioids *because they do not know what else to do.*

If we allow ourselves to become distressed or despondent about someone's suffering, it will probably not help us to help them and may add to their distress. But we are human and are bound to react in this way sometimes. Should we always try to suppress this? The alternative, detachment, can be an effective way of protecting ourselves and ensuring that our judgement remains rational and objective, but if the patient perceives us to be detached, may this only add to the common experience of feeling abandoned? Might it make them feel a little better if we frankly admit our frustration and openly share some of their distress? Traditionally the response to this problem has simply been seen as steering a course between the Scylla of over-involvement and the Charybidis of detachment, but the recognition of acceptance as something potentially positive has added new complexities, challenges and opportunities. The skills of exploring, meeting and using these cannot be easily taught, may take a professional lifetime to learn and mistakes will still be all too frequent. They depend on finding a common language to share with the patient which may be different for each individual. Realistic expectation must be balanced with hope, and authority with empathy. The process of encouraging acceptance requires sensitivity and time, and may even need to be started at the first consultation. It is important to stress that acceptance is not the same as pessimism, nor even resignation, and above all is not a road that the patient will have to travel alone.

A GLOBAL CONTEXT

So far our discussion of acceptance has been relatively parochial and applicable only where a full range of pain management services is available including biomedicine, psychology and other healing arts. But suffering is universal. When we look at the world beyond our shores, poverty and hunger, often exacerbated by conflict or natural disaster, are at least as prolific sources of suffering as disease, injury and pain. So many people seem to be denied the most basic medical needs, let alone any sophisticated pain management. By our standards the treatment of pain is often so woefully inadequate that millions of people would appear to be experiencing unrelenting suffering. But if your experience is that this has always been the case and apparently always will be, do you accept it? If people who share your culture appear to accept suffering, do you accept it too? If your religion teaches that suffering is the will of God or the inescapable consequence of your karma, does that help you to accept it? Does that make it easier to bear? Can you be happy in the face of poverty, hunger and disease if you accept it? We often see pictures of people who certainly appear to be happy in conditions that we would find intolerable. Gordon Waddell pointed out years ago that the epidemic of disability from back pain we have witnessed in affluent countries was simply non-existent in those where there are no unemployment or sickness benefits, and where you either work or starve, although there is no reason at all to assume that there is any less back pain. Are there then different standards of acceptability for us and for them? We can only hope that the answers to these questions may at least sometimes be yes, for all the hope of the situation ever changing for the better. In October 2004, the International Association for the Study of Pain (ISAP) and the European Federation of IASP Chapters, together with the World Health Organization, declared that pain relief should be a universal human right; a noble intention which should prioritise the addressing of huge unfulfilled needs in both the developed and developing world. Nevertheless in a world of so many conflicting priorities (which in too many countries include the provision of the most basic medical care) some doubt is bound to arise regarding the realism of such a proposal.

Although we cannot pretend that we live in isolation and have no responsibilities towards poorly resourced countries, we have to be very careful how we institute and carry this out. Developing countries would unquestionably be better off with more readily available technical resources but if these are not introduced as part of a country's culture their overall effect may be damaging. We live in times where health provisions can vary immensely within a country depending on ability to pay for treatment. The monetary gap between the world's richest and poorest is widening; corruption, greed, unemployment and poverty are at an all-time high. We may argue that poverty, hunger and disease are the responsibility of governments and non-governmental organisations, but pain practitioners in the affluent world surely also have responsibilities, particularly as regards education (the IASP has indeed made considerable progress in facilitating education about pain medicine in developing countries) and acceptance of the apparent inevitability of all the suffering in the world emphatically does not let us off the hook of facing these.

CONCLUSION: RESOLVING PARADOXES?

The last paragraph may seem somewhat removed from learning acceptance in the context of the pain clinic, but I think the same potential conflict between acceptance of suffering and our obligation to do something about it pertains. I believe that it involves the same intellectual and emotional processes by which we struggle to reconcile and cope with this and the many other paradoxes which face us every day. I suspect it is something we will never completely resolve.

FURTHER READING

➤ Bowker J. *Problems of Suffering in Religions of the World*. Cambridge: Cambridge University Press; 1970.

Index